OWN YOUR HEALTH: *Healthy to 100*

OWN YOUR HEALTH

The Best of Alternative & Conventional Medicine

Healthy to 100

AGING WITH VIGOR AND GRACE

ALEXA FLECKENSTEIN, M.D. AND ROANNE WEISMAN

Health Communications, Inc.
Deerfield Beach, Florida

www.hcibooks.com

This book is not intended to be a substitute for the advice and/or medical care of the reader's physician. The reader should consult with a physician in all matters related to his or her health.

Library of Congress Cataloging-in-Publication Data
available from the Library of Congress

Publisher: Health Communications, Inc.
            3201 S.W. 15th Street
            Deerfield Beach, FL 33442–8190

Cover and inside book design by Lawna Patterson Oldfield
Cover photos ©Artville, ©Shutterstock

CONTENTS

   Aches and Pains • Alzheimer's Disease •
   Arthritis • Cellulite • Chronic Bronchitis,
   COPD, Respiratory Disease • Chronic Pain •
   Colds and Flu • Constipation • Depression •
   Diabetes • Dizziness, Frequent Falls, Loss of
   Balance, Vertigo • Eye Problems • Fatigue,
   Daytime Sleepiness, Chronic Weakness • Gout •
   Hair Loss • Heartburn, GERD, Reflux, Dyspepsia,
   Stomach Pain, Gastritis • Heart Disease •
   Hemorrhoids • High Blood Pressure • High
   Cholesterol • Hot Flashes and Other Menopausal
   Symptoms • Impotence, Loss of Desire and

Missing Orgasms (in Women) • Incontinence,
Urinary (Women) • Insomnia • Liver Spots •
Memory Loss • Osteoporosis • Overweight,
Obesity • Pain • Parkinson's Disease • Prostate
Ailments • Smoking (Quitting) • Stress • Stroke
• Thyroid Disease • Ulcers (Skin), Pressure
Ulcers • Urinary Tract Infection (UTI) • Vaginal
Dryness and Itching After Menopause • Varicose
Veins • Wrinkles

PREFACE

To me, "owning my health" means taking as much responsibility as possible for what goes on in my body. It is the opposite of feeling like the helpless victim of pain, disease or disability. It also means working in a collaborative partnership with my doctor to find the best ways to prevent and treat disease from all worlds of medicine: alternative and complementary, as well as conventional.

Here is how I learned to "own my health": In 1995, I woke up from heart-valve surgery with the left side of my body paralyzed from a stroke. A tiny piece of tissue had broken away from the valve, traveled through blood vessels and lodged in my brain, blocking the flow of blood with its essential supply of oxygen to the neurons that controlled movement on my left side.

If I had obediently followed the prescribed role of stroke patient in the world of conventional medicine, I would be dependent on adaptive devices and other people for many of the activities of daily life. Instead, I have recovered completely and am back to my life as a medical journalist, wife and mother.

I quickly learned that while the advances of modern medicine can save your life, the conventional medical system—along with the insurers who pay for it—is not set up for true healing. The goal of the system was to get me to a minimal level of functioning, out of the hospital or rehabilitation facility and back home. What happened after that was up to me.

As a patient, it often feels as if the conventional health-care system wants us to accept and "adapt" to our health problems—whether we are recovering from a heart attack or stroke or suffering from chronic illness or pain. We often feel as if we are being treated as collections of body parts to be "fixed" with pills or adaptive devices, rather than as whole people with emotions, relationships, minds and spirits.

By contrast, "integrative medicine," which is the philosophy of this *Own Your Health* book series, encourages people to combine complementary and alternative medicine (often called "CAM") with conventional medicine to find true healing of body, mind and spirit—to achieve wholeness.

As we grow older, we often feel particularly alone in the world of conventional medicine. In her Introduction to this book, Dr. Alexa Fleckenstein, a board-certified internist with a sub-specialty in European Natural Medicine, shares with us many of the fears that her patients have voiced about growing older. These include pain, loss of function, depression, loneliness and fear of catastrophic illness. From her perspective of more than two decades of medical practice, Dr. Fleckenstein assures us, however, that growing older can be blissful. She guides us in how to listen to the wisdom of our bodies, engage in healthy living, and make use of complementary and alternative health systems as well as conventional medicine. And, she tells us, no matter what your age, it is never too soon or too late to start preparing for a long, healthy, vigorous life.

Going outside of the conventional medical system can be a tough thing to do for those of us who are accustomed to seeing our doctors as omniscient beings who control our health, but with Dr. Fleckenstein's guidance, you will learn about many effective options for aging with vigor and grace. When I looked for ways to expand my own healing options, I found treatments that helped me both recover movement and reduce pain. These included acupuncture and tai chi from the ancient system of Traditional Chinese Medicine; yoga, from the equally ancient Indian Ayurvedic system of medicine; the Alexander Technique—a powerful system of movement education that teaches you to use your body with less effort and reduced pain; craniosacral therapy; and various forms of bodywork and massage.

In addition to these healing methods, Dr. Fleckenstein shares easy ways to incorporate nutritional changes, exercise and joy into a lifestyle that promotes longevity and good health—adding life to your years and years to your life. I am grateful that Dr. Fleckenstein of WholeHealth New England, an integrative medical practice, is the coauthor of this book. She will be a wonderful "travel guide" on your journey toward "owning your health" and a healthy and vigorous long life.

—*Roanne Weisman*

INTRODUCTION

*One sees a flame in the eyes
of the young, but in the eyes of
the old, one sees light.*

—Victor Hugo

When I was seventeen, I thought how absolutely devastating it must be to grow old—twenty-five, for example—and not to dance to rock and roll every night. By 25 I was a mother (probably as a direct consequence of having danced to rock-and roll-every night. . . .) and had developed a different set of interests and values. I had made new friends and had a new life. Rock and roll was still fun—but only occasionally.

Are you afraid of getting older? In a society that puts much emphasis on youth, getting older can be scary. Hitting forty or fifty, or any other round number that you do not even want to whisper to yourself, can pull the rug out from under your feet. You feel as if you are losing your balance—sometimes physically as well as emotionally—and you have to find a new center for each new stage of life: children leaving home, the end of a career, the loss of some physical function, a change in your relationship with your spouse, losses and bereavements of all kinds.

Here are some fears of getting older that my patients have shared with me:

- Never having the chance to live the life of my dreams
- Losing my marbles
- Being unable to care for myself
- Being sexually unattractive/never having sex again
- Becoming homeless
- Never finding a partner
- Being unable to keep my present partner
- Never having the children I always wanted
- Dying without having grandchildren
- Being put on the "invisible shelf"—feeling useless to society
- Running out of money
- Never resolving family feuds

- Having to care for aging relatives
- Fearing God's wrath because I've lost my belief
- Being alone and lonely
- Leaving my partner alone and lonely
- Becoming a burden to my children
- Suffering pain and agony in my final illness

It seems that people fear that the end of life—loneliness, decrepitude, pain, poverty, powerlessness might come before death. But it does not have to be that way! You have the potential to design your future, and this book will help you take your health and your future into your own hands.

Many of those who have visited that scary place of older age assure us that getting older can be blissful—especially if you consider the alternative. I was a sickly child who nearly died of tuberculosis at age twelve. Now, as a physician, mother and grandmother, I cherish the many birthdays behind me! I have learned to savor every moment and every day of living. I learned that you have to be fully alive until you are dead, or life is wasted. Getting older is only frightening if you think that being seventeen is the pinnacle of life. It is not.

On the other hand, don't think that your fears will vanish like ice in the sun. To live a full life and to age successfully means you have to face your fears—and still do what you want to do or what needs to be done.

In this book you won't find "dramatic break-throughs" or the latest concoction in a bottle. We don't vie for your money—only for your attention. We offer common-sense advice and methods that are tried and true as well as supported by the newest research.

Think of this book as your travel guide through the adventure of getting older. We will talk about the attitudes you will "pack" for this important journey, the food that will nourish you, the discoveries you will make, and the activities that will help invigorate your body and soul. Along the way, we will combine modern medical science with the healing traditions—some of them ancient—of other cultures around the world. You will learn how easy it is to incorporate health-promoting practices seamlessly into your everyday life.

The fact that you are reading a book in the *Own Your Health* series shows that you are ready to take responsibility for your health—no matter which "big birthday" you are facing next. You are obviously curious about learning, growth and change, and are ready to make that first step to being healthy to 100. It is never too soon or too late to begin invigorating your body and soul!

The Wisdom of Age

Older folks have always attracted me. When I was four years old in postwar Europe, we lived in an art-deco villa that had served as the home of one family before the war; now thirteen families were living in its thirteen rooms. While my parents were working, they left me with an elderly neighbor in the basement. I called her "Auntie," even if she was just one of the strangers that the turbulent times had thrown together. Auntie worked as a seamstress; her sewing machine clattered all day long. I was proud that I could help her thread her needles, which was difficult for her because of her diminished eyesight. I looked at her wrinkled, benevolent face and asked myself how it must feel to be so old and to have survived so much heartbreak.

Auntie's stories about her life fascinated me. Before the war, she had been a photographer and had owned a shop—at a time when few women owned businesses. On the wall hung a large framed photo of a young, blonde girl, full of life and expectations—her daughter. She had died in the big flu epidemic of 1919 at the age of fourteen. I mourned that beautiful girl, but what I really wanted to know was how one could survive such a calamity and still be in one piece.

During the past two decades, I have cared for thousands of adult patients, many of them elderly. The older ones always put a spell on me because if they had made it that far, they had interesting stories to tell, and I loved to listen to them. Where else but in the stories of the people who have been there can a young person get a glimpse of how to survive divorce, war, the death of a child or a spouse, displacement and life-threatening illness?

I remember one patient, Dorothy. She was in her seventies and had been diagnosed with severe heart disease and narrowing of the arteries to her brain. All of her doctors, including me, recommended surgery. But Dorothy refused. Instead of being in despair, she asked me, "What can I do to reverse this disease?" I worried about her not having surgery, but I respected her decision. And I thought that with her upbeat attitude, Dorothy had a good chance. We worked together, following many of the principles you will learn in this book. Now, years later, she is doing fine. "I am walking better," she told me just the other day. "I have more energy. I handle stress better. My health is improving all the time."

Two things that older people say when they open up always strikes me: "I still feel like a five-year-old discovering the world. I can't believe this is me," and "Memories from the past are not distant and gone. It seems that everything I experienced in my life is with me right now." These two sentiments reflect both the joy of new discoveries and an appreciation of the lessons learned from the past—both essential components of a life well lived.

THE INTEGRATIVE APPROACH TO GROWING OLDER

Your body is designed to heal itself and find the balance of health that is right for you. Tapping into this healing ability is especially important when facing chronic illness or pain that often accompany growing older. We all have innate capacities to restore balance, repair damaged cells and recover from illness. Problems arise when these natural healing abilities are blocked, either by stress, poor diet or a lifestyle that demands too much of us. Conventional medicine is good at diagnosing certain diseases and treating the symptoms of acute illness and injury. At times, the conventional medical approach is clearly the right answer.

However, it is less effective at helping to stimulate our own natural healing abilities and less focused on treating the whole person.

Integrative medicine, on the other hand, recognizes that we are more than the cells, molecules and atoms that make up our bodies. We all have something else—something that won't show up on an X-ray or CT scan. We can call this our life force, "Qi" (pronounced "chi"), spirit, energy or many other names. But whatever we call it, it is this intangible "energy" that heals. It empowers our immune system so that our bodies can repair damage from the stress, bacteria, viruses, pollution, injuries and other onslaughts that most of us deal with every day. The Consortium for Academic Health Centers for Integrative Medicine recently defined integrative medicine as "the practice of medicine that reaffirms the importance of relationship between practitioner and patient, focuses on the whole person, is informed by evidence, and makes use of all appropriate therapeutic approaches to achieve optimal health and healing."

The Importance of "Owning Your Health" Throughout Life

"Your health is in your hands," says Ester R. Shapiro, Ph.D. "Although you may not have control of the course of an illness, how you respond to that illness—drawing on the support of family, community, your own beliefs and spiritual values—can help you heal." A psychologist, researcher, writer and teacher, Shapiro notes that only approximately ten percent of health outcomes are produced by any contact with the health system. As much as 90 percent are due to your lifestyle, economic resources, social support, and a sense of power in determining the course and condition of your life and the lives of your family and community. Research shows that people who feel a sense of control—of ownership—of their health do better clinically than those who feel that they are helpless victims of their illness. Shapiro's writing and work focus on the way in which people and their families deal with extraordinary life challenges, including pain, illness and death.[1] In our book, you will learn ways to build the resilience, good health and vitality that will carry you through the prime of your life with joy and vigor.

1

WHAT CAN WE LEARN FROM PEOPLE WHO LIVE TO BE 100?

Y ou and I are mere youngsters compared to the more than 100 people in New England who have passed their 100th birthdays and are participating in the New England Centenarian Study (NECS), a joint project of Boston Medical Center and the Harvard Medical School, founded and directed by geriatrics expert Thomas T. Perls, M.D., M.P.H. The study, which started in 1994, is the first comprehensive investigation of the world's oldest people.

While the research does seem to indicate a link between genetics and longevity, lifestyle also plays an important role in both the quality of life and the quantity of years. As one expert has said, "It's not just your genes; it's what you do with them." In presenting the findings of their research, Perls and colleague Margery Hutter Silver, M.D., make it clear that even if you don't have the "extreme age" gene, it is possible to live a full, long, healthy life by following the examples of those who have done just that. "We look at aging as an opportunity rather than a curse," says Perls.

In their book, *Living to 100, Lessons in Living to Your Maximum Potential at Any Age*, Perls and Silver describe several centenarians who have reached extreme old age in good health, exploding the myth that aging has to be associated with disease and deterioration.

What do all centenarians have in common? Well, for starters, they don't set out to become that old; they just live one day at a time and enjoy it. The following section lists what else they share.

Best Ways to Live a Long, Healthy Life: Do What Centenarians Do

According to the New England Centenarian Study, people who have passed their 100th birthdays may have the genes to help them, but they also have lifestyles that are remarkably similar:[2]

- Healthy centenarians stay connected with others of all age groups and involved in their communities.
- They keep physically active with regular, daily exercise. They bake and cook for family gatherings, go to the office and play golf. One woman, 101 years old, has a habit of reading while riding a stationary bicycle.
- They continue to use their brains throughout their lives. Many experts recommend learning new skills as a way to keep the brain functioning. Try a new language!
- They have learned how to handle stress and the many losses that happen on the way to 100.[3]
- They use humor to cope with difficult times. "He who laughs, lasts," says Perls.
- They find meaning in some kind of spiritual practice and seem to take a lively interest and joy in everything around them.

I would add to this list that the extremely old people whom I have met in my practice are self-sufficient—they remain living independently as long as possible, they adapt well to challenges, they have good sleep habits, regular bowel movements, and prefer outdoor activities and fresh air. *Centenarians focus on living each day as it comes instead of on living a long time*. Being old is not different from being young—except in one important way: People fail all the time at being young, making lousy decisions and not learning anything new. Old people, by contrast, have made at least some good decisions—otherwise they could not have survived so long.

Centenarians are not always nice; some are cantankerous and ornery. Most of them have been married, and most have been widowed. But after their losses, they grieved and got over it. Most are women—many of whom, interestingly, have borne children after their fortieth birthdays. The most prominent trait that centenarians have in common, though, is their self-sufficiency. Many eschew pills, unless they are absolutely necessary.

The Importance of Resilience and Hardiness[4]

Twenty-five years ago, psychologist Salvatore R. Maddi, Ph.D., asked himself: "Why do some people suffer physical and mental breakdowns when faced with overwhelming stress while others seem to thrive?" At that time, Dr. Maddi was studying creativity. "I was learning that creative people—such as artists, writers, musicians or theatrical professionals—are always looking for new experiences and new answers to questions," says Dr. Maddi. Other people, by contrast, become debilitated and even ill in response to stressful changes in their lives.

Dr. Maddi's interest in people's different responses to stress spurred him to take his research in a new direction, and he began looking for a sample of highly stressed people. He found them at Illinois Bell Telephone (IBT), where he was working as a consultant. "Due to the 1981 deregulation of the telephone industry, IBT downsized from 26,000 employees to just over half that many in one year," says Dr. Maddi. "The remaining employees faced changing job descriptions, company goals and supervisors. One manager reported having ten different supervisors in one year."

Dr. Maddi and his group evaluated the IBT employees during a landmark twelve-year study. On a yearly basis for the six years before the deregulation and downsizing, Dr. Maddi and his research team used complex and in-depth psychological and medical measuring tools to study more than 400 supervisors, managers and executives at IBT. After the downsizing, they were able to continue following the original study group on a yearly basis until 1987.

"We found that about two-thirds of the employees in the study suffered significant performance, leadership and health declines—including heart attacks, strokes, obesity, depression, substance abuse and poor performance reviews—as the result of the extreme stress in their workplace," says Dr. Maddi. "However, the other one-third actually thrived during the upheaval, despite experiencing the same amount of disruption and stressful events as their co-workers. These employees maintained their health, happiness and performance and felt renewed enthusiasm." The differences between the two groups prior to the upheaval led Dr. Maddi to identify the concept of *hardiness*.[5] "The research revealed that those who thrived during stressful times had maintained three key beliefs that helped them turn adversity into an advantage. We call these beliefs 'The Three Cs of Hardiness,'" says Dr. Maddi. According to his research, hardiness moderates the relationship between stress and illness and can act as a "buffer" against stress-related illnesses, even when people have inherited vulnerability to such illnesses.[6]

Dr. Maddi's Three Cs of Hardiness:
Commitment, Control and Challenge

Three hardiness attitudes, which Dr. Maddi calls "The Three Cs," increase resilience and hardiness. They may also lead to a longer, healthier life. These three attitudes are *commitment, control* and *challenge*. Dr. Maddi points out that later studies show hardiness to be roughly two times as effective in decreasing the subsequent risk of illness as social support and physical exercise.[7]

Commitment. The commitment attitude leads people to strive to be involved with people, things and contexts rather than being detached, isolated or alienated.

Control. The control attitude leads people to struggle to have an influence on the outcomes going on around themselves, rather than lapsing into passivity and powerlessness.

Challenge. The challenge attitude leads people to learn continually from their experiences, viewing acute and chronic stresses, whether positive or negative, as opportunities for new learning. Hardy people do not "play it safe" by avoiding uncertainties and potential threats. Rather, they are motivated by challenges to learn how they can grow and change for the better.

Most important for our purposes, Dr. Maddi's research and extensive clinical work demonstrate that you can learn to acquire and use hardy attitudes, even if you were not born with a hardy disposition.[8] Hardiness training programs enhance performance, leadership, stamina, mood, and both physical and mental health by giving people the courage and capability to turn adversity into advantage.[9]

HEALTHY TO 100 TIP

George Bernard Shaw once said, "Youth is wasted on the young." Why is that so? Because young people live in the future, with all their dreams and plans, and they don't see the wonderful life around them. Don't give up your dreams and your plans, but live today and enjoy the here and now. You never know how much future you will have.

You might still want to achieve some long-cherished goals, but it doesn't have to be all toil and sweat. Reaching 100 is not a competition. You have nothing to prove. By grace, you may one day get there—but it is not worthwhile if you didn't have fun on the way. Relax and take one day at a time.

"Don't Fence Me In":
A Portrait of Jinny

If you are curious about what resilience and hardiness look like, meet Jinny, who describes herself as an extrovert. "I like to connect with people. In Jungian terms, I like to imprint myself on my environment."

Here is Jinny's environment: She lives alone with two golden cats in a sunny apartment with pots of herbs and plants thriving on window ledges; a treadmill (for when she can't get out to exercise); a study lined with floor-to-ceiling bookshelves displaying her passions for gourmet cooking, Jungian psychology, art, music and architectural history; and paintings, wall hangings, prints, sculptures, maps and drawings from all over the world, gathered in her travels. "I have met almost all the people whose art I have," she says. "I would have loved to have known Rembrandt, but I can't afford him anyway."

Jinny spends her summers in a rental cottage in Maine, swimming regularly in the frigid ocean. "It is very stimulating," she says. "I can spend about fifteen minutes thrashing around and come out looking like a cooked lobster. I believe seawater is therapeutic: The ocean is the mother of us all." During the summer, she also works out three times a week at a nearby health club.

During the spring and fall, Jinny walks twenty-five minutes every week to her community garden plot. (She sold her car long ago and walks or takes public transportation everywhere.) On this early spring day, she has just planted her peas, lugging forty pounds of topsoil in a grocery cart up the hill. When she first got the garden ten years ago, she spent eight hours "double-digging" down eighteen inches to aerate it. "I did it in two-hour shifts," she says. This spring, as usual, she will fertilize it with cow manure and topsoil as well as with minerals and fertilizer that she orders during the winter. When she needs help with transportation, a friend with a neighboring plot drives her. "She offered to be my chauffeur if I'd be her gardening guru," says Jinny. This year, she plans to grow her usual crops, including rhubarb, herbs, potatoes, tomatoes, egg-plant, lettuces, beets, carrots, onions, arugula and tiny wild strawberries.

Did we mention that Jinny was born in 1915? No matter. It hardly seems relevant. "I guess I'm still a child at heart," she says. When interviewed three years ago, she was already planning her ninetieth birthday party: "It will be a dance party with a jazz combo," she said at the time. "Stick around." This year, Jinny had the party she had been dreaming of, with not one but *two* jazz combos, and plenty of dancing and food for all of her friends and family.

Full of as much vigor as ever at ninety, Jinny is still swimming and gardening. She has regular shiatsu massages and osteopathic treatments, practices yoga and continues her twice-weekly workouts at a Pilates studio. "All of this keeps things moving and aligned," she says.

When she's not moving her body, she coordinates volunteers at a local university's "Learning in Retirement" program, where she also co-teaches a course in analytical psychology and takes classes. She listens to the Metropolitan Opera on the radio and cooks herself a gourmet dinner most evenings. "Last night, I made golden beets with beet greens, a mélange of red peppers, okra, zucchini, onion and garlic, cooked in olive oil, served over gemelli pasta," she says. "I also like lamb and pork, but mostly fish."

Jinny has had only two major health problems in her long life: "When I was in my sixties I had pneumonia, and it took me about a year to get my energy back," she says. "Then my knee began bothering me when I was eighty-three, and I needed to use a cane. An arthroscopy didn't help, so I had the whole joint replaced. After a few months, I was better than ever!"

Divorced twice and the mother of two, Jinny has been an amateur actress and a faculty wife, and has traveled extensively, living for a time in Costa Rica during World War II with her first husband and two small children. After her first divorce, she lived with her children in Washington, D.C., managed a bookstore and sold real estate. During and after her second marriage, she lived in Illinois and New York City, studied fine arts at NYU, became certified as a graphologist (handwriting expert) and began what was to become a lifelong study of Jungian psychology at the C. G. Jung Foundation. She also became director of a committee providing service and information to United Nations delegations. "All of my life, I have refused to be tied down," she says. "Don't fence me in."

2

EXAMINE YOUR
ATTITUDES

You cannot do anything about getting older every minute. But you can get wiser and better and grow all the time. Then suddenly age is fun. If you resist change, on the other hand, aging will become your misery. The day you learn to laugh about yourself, you become *wise*.

One way to become wise is to travel *inside* yourself and explore your attitudes, feelings, emotions and the ways in which past experiences are still affecting you—even if you are not aware of it.

One of the best ways to take this inward journey is by sharing your deepest emotions and thoughts, either in writing or in talking with others. Dr. James W. Pennebaker is professor of psychology at the

University of Texas at Austin, where he and his students are exploring the links between traumatic experiences and physical and mental health.[10] His studies find that physician use, medical costs and alcohol consumption can be reduced and work performance increased by simple writing and/or talking exercises. His most recent research focuses on the nature of language and emotion in the real world. "Writing about emotional upheavals in our lives can improve physical and mental health," says Dr. Pennebaker. "Keep in mind that there are probably a thousand ways to write that may be beneficial to you," he says. "Experiment on your own and see what works best."[11]

Recently, a participant in one of our *Own Your Health* workshops described how she starts a new journal every year on her birthday, after rereading the journal from the previous year. She clearly owns her year. It might be fun to buy your own beautiful journal in which to record the dreams you have at night, your thoughts during the day, your memories of traumatic events in your life, and begin to see what patterns emerge from your "inner landscape." But until you do, why not begin jotting some thoughts down here?

_____

_____

_____

_____

_____

_____

You *can* reach for goals and dreams, even if you already have some life travel behind you. A new career, a better partnership, a healthier body, a more fulfilled life—they all are still possible. Anything is possible. You can do it if you think you can. Believe in yourself, and begin your new life today.

Before you die, what do you want to have accomplished?

_____

_____

_____

_____

Do you want to leave your house in order? Make a long journey? Reconnect with a lost friend or your alienated sister? Do you want to find your spiritual path? Do you want to leave your present life and do what you have felt for a long time you must be doing? Do you want to take up pottery or work in an auto shop? Go for a camel ride in the desert? What are you waiting for? Get started today!

What do you want be said about you at your funeral or in your obituary? This is a painful but important exercise because it can help you determine what is truly important in your life, and what your purpose on this Earth might be.

_____

_____

_____

_____

_____

_____

Keeping the Mind Alive— While Having Fun! A Portrait of Danny

One of the notable findings of aging research is the mental and physical health benefit of lifelong learning—of keeping the mind active. You can do it as Jinny does, by taking courses and listening to opera. But if that is not to your taste, there is always poker.

Danny is seventy-seven years old, and he's been an avid poker player for most of his life. He has the quiet smile of people who have lived a contented life. "I've always been good with numbers," he says. He loves doing calculations in his head and will cheerfully put you to a challenge: "I bet I can add up a column of numbers in my head faster than you can with a calculator," he says roguishly. He's right.

For Danny, exercising his mind, either with arithmetic or with poker, is a lifelong hobby. He is still as mentally sharp as he was thirty years ago. One of the owners of a bead-importing business, he goes to the office four days a week and plays golf on the weekends. But his real passion is poker. "I play two or three times a week," he says. For Danny, poker is serious business. "During a game, I am thinking and strategizing with every turn of the cards," he says. "I calculate percentages and odds, my position at the table and the amount to bet or raise. It is exciting, a real adrenalin rush. I get so charged up that I can easily play for six or seven hours!"

Danny also likes the social aspects of the game. "One of my regular games has been going on with many of the same guys every Monday night for thirty years." While he enjoys playing with friends, he also likes the challenge of poker tournaments. "These are not my friends, but I love the competition," he says. "It keeps the mind alive."

If you still strive for a better you, then you are not really old. It can be something as easy as filling out a crossword puzzle. Or learning square dance, lumberjacking, paintball or bridge. You might find they are not for you, but from there, you go on learning something else. The new challenge keeps you alive and young at heart. You keep your mental capacities by applying them: *Use it or lose it.*

3

THE COURAGE
TO CHANGE

If you don't believe that it is possible to completely change your life, listen to this: In Germany, I had an older friend, who, in her mid-fifties, began psychotherapy because she could not stand the person she had been all her life. In her youth, she had been an enthusiastic follower of Hitler. After the war, she found herself a prostitute, then a lousy mother for her children and a cold wife to her older husband, whom she had married for convenience. She would drink at parties and say unkind and spiteful things to people. She judged herself superficial, untruthful, cruel and craving attention.

In therapy, she began to excavate long-buried feelings about her past and its damaging effects on her personality. She had been an orphan tossed around by unloving relatives and had been sexually abused by several uncles. With this newfound awareness and connection to her past, she found the energy to make dramatic changes in her life. She cared for her ailing husband until he died, trying to make up for her previous cruelty. She started a job that rewarded her with new insights and new acquaintances. She consciously avoided people who brought out the worst in her. She forged new and loving friendships and went on a quest that brought her into the theater as an extra. That suited her flamboyant personality and her need for attention. She learned meditation and yoga, and she built a sauna in her tiny apartment with what little money she had. In everything, she faced her bad sides with honesty. She died twenty-five years later, a woman finally at peace with herself. I will not give you her name because I want to protect her family, but she was one of my best friends ever.

In essence, my friend found out who she was and what she needed. The more honest she became with herself and her surroundings, the more things happened to make her happy, and the better a person she became.

HEALTHY TO 100 TIP

Here are my suggestions for positive change:

- Live with an attitude of gratitude.
- Use therapy, journal writing or talking to close friends to understand yourself and your relationship to the past.
- Make friends, cherish neighbors, keep in touch with family.
- Build a network of supportive people. Don't go it alone.
- Talk openly about the problems and hardships you have because nobody can help you if they don't know you need help.
- Stop complaining and take action instead.
- Don't use age as an excuse to accept your situation. It is never too late to improve. Leave your old fears behind and try something new today!
- Try to find role models who lived with spunk, vigor and compassion. I always think of Eleanor Roosevelt, but perhaps you have your own "heroes."

I recall a story about a patient who in his early sixties was admitted to the hospital with heart failure. He was restored, given a lot of pills and sent home with the advice to take it easy and prepare for his death. The man threw out the pills, changed some eating habits, and returned to the rose garden that was his passion. He lived another 25 years. Because he had something he loved.

Not to be tried at home, of course—he could have died without his medication. But still, I love the story and the spunk of the man. By the way, he died in his rose garden.

Give to Yourself by Giving to Others

When I grew up after World War II in Germany, I did not know a single interesting woman. My beautiful mother and her beautiful girlfriends all acted as if thirty were over the hill, and forty was the end of life, dreaded more than death. When one of her best friends died in a car accident at forty, my mother pronounced her the "luckiest girl in the world." Suicide was seriously contemplated. I decided I never wanted to be as shallow and self-centered.

In the past several years, researchers have shown that serving other people in the community might have a positive influence on health or well-being not only for the recipient of service, but also for the provider of service.[12] One study, reported by Tiffany

Field, Ph.D., director of the Touch Research Institute, asked elderly people to act as volunteer "grandparents." "Elderly people are noted to suffer from touch deprivation," wrote Field. The study, which recruited volunteer "grandparents" and trained them to give infant massage, hypothesized that the massage interaction would benefit both infant and "grandparent," and that is exactly what happened.

During a one-month period of massaging infants, the volunteer "grandparents" experienced increased self-esteem, decreased levels of cortisol (a stress hormone), and improvements in their lifestyles. They also reported drinking less coffee, making more social contacts and fewer visits to the doctor. Interestingly, reports Field, in a second part of the study, elderly volunteers benefited more from *giving* massages to infants than from *receiving* professional massages themselves.[13]

The benefits received from giving occur not only from physical services or gifts, but also when we give mentally and spiritually: for example, when we pray for others. In one study, people who prayed for others scored significantly better on objective measures of self-esteem, anxiety and depression than did the people they prayed for.

The people who did the praying also reported reduced anxiety, improved mood, reduced illness symptoms and lowered depression.[14]

Find Your Creative Purpose in Life

Every person has a deep purpose in life—each of us has been put on this Earth for a reason. Create a life for yourself around that purpose! Deepak Chopra, in his *Ageless Body, Timeless Mind* says: "I am more than my atoms, they come and go."[15] The molecules and atoms in your body are constantly exchanged—it is estimated that in about seven years every single atom of your body is turned over and replaced. That turnover of cells, of course, is your chance to build a better body with better nutrition and exercise—but it won't change the eternal spirit living in you. That spirit is part of the universe—eternally joyful and creative.

Because you are unique, take a moment every day and make it your quiet time. Native Americans used to greet the dawning sun alone—to be reminded every day of the scheme of things. But you can take "your" time anytime: a lone walk of a few minutes at lunch break, a few minutes of meditation and relaxation in the car in the driveway before you brace for the demands and joys of your family, or withdraw into cross-stitching or wood-working.

Affirming Life with Creativity: A Portrait of Lilllian

Along a hallway of the Laurelmead Retirement Residence, you will see four large windows displaying colorful and whimsical scenes. Each of the stained-glass windows beautifully illustrates a folktale from a different cultural tradition: "The Magic Brocade" is a story of courage from ancient China. "The King with the Dirty Feet," from India, is about creativity and the invention of shoes. From Africa comes the story of "Kimwaki and the Weaver Birds," teaching a lesson about cooperation and friendliness. "Meshka, the Kvetch (complainer)" comes from Russia, and tells the story of a woman who learned to see the beauty in life rather than her own miseries.

All of the windows are low enough to be seen from a wheelchair, and each window has a comfortable chair next to it, along with a plastic frame holding the text of the folktale (in easy-to-read large print). "It feels good to see people from the nursing home being wheeled along the hallway, looking at the windows, and either reading the stories or having the attendants read to them," says Lillian in her melodious voice. She is a petite woman of eighty-two with a light step, deft hands and bright hazel eyes that seem permanently crinkled into a smile.

It is Lillian's artistry and imagination that has transformed this hallway into a place of joy, hope and optimism. Almost as soon as she and her husband, Paul, moved into the complex, she began her stained-glass project, teaching a group of residents to work with her. Before they begin work on each window, Lillian and the group of residents select the folktale, discuss it and begin to draw illustrations. When they agree on the images to include, Lillian incorporates the ideas into designs that are feasible for cut-glass shapes. "Some people cut the glass, others wrap the edges of each piece in copper foil, and then we solder the pieces together," says Lillian. "It is truly a group effort."

Lillian did not discover her creative abilities until she was sixty-five years old. "Both my father and grandfather were talented amateur artists," she says. "But I was too busy raising three children and volunteering to think about art!" Her life in stained glass began fifteen years ago with a snowstorm and a broken window. "We were shoveling a huge mound of snow in front of our house when a handle flew off a shovel and cracked one of the leaded-glass panes at our front door," she remembers. "I was wondering how we were going to get it fixed when I happened to see an advertisement in the newspaper for a stained-glass course at a nearby senior center."

Lillian signed up for the class. She soon realized that it was not technical enough to teach her how to repair the thick leaded glass at their house, but by then she was hooked. In the years that followed, she continued to create her own fanciful designs, began to teach classes in the technique, and built windows of ever-increasing beauty and complexity. Many of her windows now decorate her neighborhood: They can be seen in the children's hospital, the library and a nearby synagogue. When she moved into the senior residence, it seemed only natural for her to use her growing skill to create stained-glass windows to brighten up the facility.

"That first class unleashed a flood of creativity in me that I never suspected," she says. "For me, working in stained glass is all about connections. There are so many interweaving links in life, and if we remain alert and receptive, even as we grow older, we can make connections with others and with our own accumulated thoughts and experiences. Working with other people to create meaningful designs has helped me realize that we do not have to be alone. Enthusiasm is catching!"

When the teachers at a local day-care center heard about the first window, they asked if they could bring the children to see it. "Now, whenever we install a new window, we invite the children and the senior residents to a special tea party and window viewing," says Lillian. "We read the folktale and talk about its meaning as we look at the window."

HEALTHY TO 100 TIP

"So many older people are angry and depressed because they are focusing on what they can no longer do, making themselves and others miserable, just like 'Meshka, the Kvetch' in the Russian folktale. I believe that it is okay to be angry and sad, as long as you are creative and patient as well: Channel that anger and sadness and create something—anything!"

—*Lillian*

4

LETTING GO OF
BAD STRESS

O nce I attended a big continuing-education
meeting for physicians. Around 1,000 doctors crowded the hotel's huge ballroom. The ses-
sions were strenuous as one speaker after the
other droned on. Even during lunch hour, classes
continued; you could bring your food and eat
while listening (just to prove that doctors are no
models for health). In the late afternoon, with
exhaustion setting in, attendance dwindled. To
keep the audience in the room, the leaders organ-
ized a raffle. You could win a medical textbook—
but only if you were present when they called out
your name. I won in one of the first passes. Of
course, I was all smiles.

My neighbor, a nice and very smart doctor from one of the Boston teaching hospitals, said: "I never win anything." I was so upset that I said: "How can you know that you won't win? If you sit with me, I cannot permit such negative thinking. Say after me: '*I, too, can win.*'" Sheepishly, she repeated my words. For me, it was not about her winning. I just could not stand the sad, giving-up attitude. She won the next book. I don't think it was magic or supernatural influence; it was just chance, after all. But why shouldn't *you* have a chance, too?

Mindful Practices

Research and experience show us time and again that unhappiness, anxiety, loneliness, anger, even lacking a sense of purpose in life have measurable, negative effects on our health. These include narrowing of blood vessels, increased blood pressure, slower wound healing, less restorative sleep and heart disease.[16] One recent study has even reported that people can die of a broken heart.[17]

A very good way to let go of stress is through such mindfulness practices as yoga, tai chi and meditation. If you don't want to start with meditation, there are many ways to become more connected to your spiritual self. Remember from chapter 1 that centenarians almost universally have some kind of spiritual belief or practice.

HEALTHY TO 100 TIP

Here are some suggestions for developing a daily practice that nourishes your spirit:

- If you find solace in a religion, attend a service or prayer group at least once every week.
- If nature is your best way to recharge, regular walks in the garden, a forest, a beach or any environment that relaxes you is good for body, mind and soul. Get out in the fresh air every day and plan an outing for the weekend.
- Take some deep, cleansing morning breaths at an open window every day.
- Take five minutes every day to sit quietly in a chair, close your eyes, turn your palms face up and simply observe your breath as it enters and leaves your body.

A CLOSER LOOK

Meditation: Ancient History, Modern Benefits

The practice of meditation has been in use for thousands of years in many cultures, including Buddhist, Ayurvedic and Taoist traditions. In this country, there have been more than thirty years of research into various meditation practices, beginning with Herbert Benson, M.D., who performed the original research on the outcomes of Transcendental Meditation (a form of concentration meditation founded by Maharishi Mahesh Yogi). Dr. Benson is perhaps best known for developing and researching the "Relaxation Response."

Meditation practices in various forms have shown health benefits: "In clinically controlled trials, mindfulness or awareness meditation has been demonstrated to effectively reduce anxiety and depression, including the condition known as post-traumatic stress; to significantly reduce chronic pain caused by a variety of medical conditions; to increase life functionality; and to reduce mood disturbance and psychiatric symptoms. Most of these outcomes were achieved with patients who had not improved with traditional medical care."[18]

THE FIVE-MINUTE MEDITATION

Here is an easy way to start meditating:

1. Choose a quiet corner.
2. Set a timer for five minutes.
3. Sit with crossed legs on the floor on a cushion or on a chair.
4. Keep your back very straight. You can use a chair with a back if needed. Imagine the top of your head touching the sky.
5. Keep your hands palms up and open on your knees.
6. Close your eyes.
7. Breathe in and out slowly. You might want to count your breaths.
8. Do not move at all except to keep your back straight.
9. Be aware of the things that come to your mind: "I feel bored. My right knee hurts." Then let them float away and bring your attention back to your breathing.
10. Pay attention to your sensations: breathing, aches, itches, fears. Let them happen and then let them float away.
11. Stop when the timer rings.

> 12. Go on with your day with renewed energy and purpose.
>
> Do *not* attempt to meditate for more than five minutes without a teacher.

5

THE POWER
OF FORGIVENESS

Resentment spoils many lives. On the journey through a healthy, happy life, it is important to let go of anger, envy, resentment, jealousy and fear. This is baggage that you don't need and that will weigh you down. Realize that other people usually are not out to hurt you. But even if they are, their bad behavior harms them much more than it could ever harm you (unless they are violent—and then you should run for your life and never look back).

Fear is what keeps you small and your heart narrow. Love expands you, so make peace with people who have hurt you.

For many years my sister and I were not on speaking terms. Finally, we realized (it was a slow and painful process) that we were continuing a pattern our parents had created for us: They had played one child against the other. Years after my parents died, we decided we could let go of the old family structure and create a new relationship. Now we connect at least once a week—across the ocean between Europe and America. I cherish my sister, her humor, her loyalty, her courage. And we, who were always so different as young girls, find out how much we have in common.

Forgiveness for Health

Many years ago, someone hurt Frederic Luskin, Ph.D. "I just couldn't get over what this friend had done," says Luskin. "Every time I thought about it, I experienced the anger and resentment all over again, including the physical symptoms that these negative emotions release. This persisted long after I had lost contact with this person. After several years of this, I suddenly realized that the person who had hurt me was having a fine life, while I was still suffering over an incident that was long in the past. Why was I doing this to myself?"

Thus was born the Stanford University Forgiveness Project, one of the largest and most important studies of forgiveness ever conducted. Luskin and his colleagues at Stanford invited two groups of bereaved families from Northern Ireland to participate in the Forgiveness Project. "We felt that this was the ultimate test," he says. "There is perhaps no worse trauma than the loss of a child, a parent or another loved one to violence."

In his book, *Forgive for Good*, Luskin describes the benefits that participants reported, which include fewer health problems, less stress, fewer physical symptoms of stress, and improvements in psychological and emotional well-being, even after devastating losses. Even *thinking* about forgiveness can make a difference, he writes: "People who imagine forgiving their offender note immediate improvement in their cardiovascular, muscular and nervous systems."[19]

The negative health effects of *not* forgiving are costly, writes Luskin: "Failure to forgive may be more important than hostility as a risk factor for heart disease. People who blame other people for their troubles have higher incidences of illnesses such as cardiovascular disease and cancers. People who imagine not forgiving someone show negative changes in blood pressure, muscle tension and immune response."[20]

Forgiveness, according to Luskin, does not mean condoning or forgetting what was done to you. "Forgiveness is the feeling of peace that merges as you take your hurt less personally, take responsibility for how you feel, and become a hero instead of a victim in the story you tell."[21] In an interview, Luskin elaborates. "Forgiveness gives you access to more positive experiences," he says. "If you think of yourself as a victim, it will take your attention away from the beauty and love around you, and this is not good for your health. Each moment of appreciation, wonder and love helps to enhance your immune system and leads to improvements in your cardiovascular health."[22]

What happens when you cannot forgive? "Every time you remind yourself of the experience that caused you pain, even if it happened years ago, your body responds by releasing stress hormones," says Luskin. "One of the effects of these hormones—which activate our ancient 'fight or flight' response, is a change in the metabolism of fat in your body. The liver produces extra cholesterol, which is sent up to your heart to protect you from bleeding in case of attack. Your heart rate speeds up, and blood is directed away from the brain and into the limbs, in case quick action is needed. Every time you activate this response system, there is a physical cost to your health."[23]

People who completed the forgiveness training experienced "reduced anger, reduced depression, reduced symptoms of stress, and greater hope and vitality," says Luskin. And according to questionnaires sent to participants months afterward, these benefits persisted. "People have the capacity to forgive, but they are not taught how," says Luskin. "In our culture, we are terrific at teaching anger, judgmental behavior and creating hostility. We are not as terrific at taking ourselves out of the center of the universe, not so terrific at hope, forgiveness or positive emotions."[24]

These skills are particularly important as people age, says Luskin. "I see two types of older people in my training programs," he says. "One group realizes that life is short, and they don't want to waste whatever time they have left in anger and negative emotions. These people are resilient and generally happy. Other people are more beaten down by life. They feel they have experienced too many insults, slights and disappointments, and they are unhappy."[25]

6

SEIZE THE JOY

Helen Nearing wrote a touching account of how her 100-year-old husband, Scott, died.[26] They had left their New York life in the thirties to live closer to nature in New England. They built their own stone house (and made a living building them for other people) and raised their own produce. They did all the work from six in the morning until noon—the rest of the day was free for enjoyment: making music, pursuing arts and writing.

Scott was active in the house and garden well into his late nineties. Around his 100th birthday, however, his health failed, and he voiced the wish to stop eating. Helen let him be. As he became weaker, he rested more and more on the sofa. Finally, he refused water, too. He died a peaceful death after a long and wonderful life. He stayed in control to the end.

It is unnecessary to approach the second half of your life with fear of death. Death will come to all of us. Prepare by getting your papers and your house in order (or leave that mess blissfully to your heirs, as my sister proposes). Read books about death and dying, like *The Tibetan Book of Living and Dying*,[27] or visit a hospice—especially if you are still light-years away from dying. There are only two important things in life: love and death. Don't fear the second—it can teach you so much. Use it as a motivation to seize the joy today.

HEALTHY TO 100 TIP

Some people don't want to face death. They want to live to their last breath without a worry. That is fine, too. Just don't sit and stare death in the face without doing something about it. At the very least, make a will and keep it in a safe place.

Here are suggestions to help you seize the joy in your life:

• **Laugh often, as the centenarians do.** And laugh with a partner. Laughter is an explosion that leads to the release of feel-good hormones into your bloodstream. You can laugh because you feel mirth—but you can also laugh in order to feel good. It goes both ways. A program for heart-failure patients at the Duke Center for Integrative Medicine[28] uses many mind-body therapies, including "laughing yoga." Here is how one participant described the experience: "Have you ever sat with a group of people and someone tells you to just laugh as hard as you can? By the end, we were roaring. That made my day. It felt real good."

The late Norman Cousins, former editor of the *Saturday Review*, wrote about fighting the crippling disease ankylosing spondylitis with humor and positive thinking. In his 1981 book *Anatomy of an Illness*, Cousins described how he used Marx Brothers films and other sources of humor to cope with pain. "I made the joyous discovery that ten minutes of genuine belly laughter had an anesthetic effect and would give me at least two hours of pain-free sleep."[29] Later in the book, he describes how he became convinced that "creativity, the will to live, hope, faith, and love have biochemical significance and contribute strongly to healing and to well-being. The positive emotions are life-giving experiences."[30]

Similarly, smiling uses many more muscles than frowning, and triggers a happiness response in your brain—even if you are not really happy. So, smile when you are alone or walking the streets; soon you might feel better.

- **Have sex.** Either with a partner or with yourself. Enjoy it. Sex is a great outlet for tension; besides that, it is a perfectly joyful way to exercise your muscles. If you have a partner, touch is a key to your well-being. If you don't have a partner, give and take as many hugs as you can get—including from your pet.

  Sex is an expression of being alive. It is a great stress reducer—unless you create stress about sex. Don't.

- Always smile at yourself in the mirror—you are your best friend.

- Find balance. Don't try to do everything right; have some fun, too. Pamper yourself occasionally with a treat (one of mine is a small piece of chocolate every few days). Don't spoil yourself with an ice cream every day—but once a month is fine (if you can handle the inevitable cravings for more).

• Appreciate little things. During an interview, a 100-year-old woman showed her visitor a photograph and said, "Today, I am particularly enjoying this photo my daughter just sent to me of a beautiful flowering plant in the desert, near where she lives." She handed over the photograph, her eyes lingering on the image of white flowers emerging from a bed of rock and sand. "Such beauty, pushing its way through the most difficult ground," she said with a smile. "What a miracle."[31]

7

LOOK GOOD,
FEEL GOOD

You don't travel in pajamas or a sweat suit. You dress up for the occasion—just as much as to show the world who you are as to meet the challenges of climate and circumstances. Looks are important.

The healthier you live, the healthier you look—it is that simple. Here are some tips:

- **Make sure you drink enough water.** I can always observe in my husband's face if he forgot to drink water; he ages immediately.
- **Sleep enough.** Nothing can smooth out wrinkles and revive a dull complexion like a good night's sleep—not to mention getting

you into a good mood. People usually need six to eight hours of sleep—and it is very individual. The best hours for repairing the immune system and body tissues are from 11 P.M. to 1 A.M.—so the old saying that sleep before midnight is the best has truth in it. (If you are having trouble sleeping, see "Insomnia" in chapter 14.)

- **Carry yourself proudly.** Slump is the most obvious sign of aging. Good posture gives a youthful impression (told to you by somebody who has to work very hard on this point). Yoga, tai chi and strength-training classes help with both balance and posture.

Wrinkles?

When I was young, somebody impressed me by saying that by the age of thirty you have the face you deserve. These are *your* wrinkles; you earned them by laughter and tears. Don't wish them away. Smile some new wrinkles into your face and get on with your day.

Sun, of course, is the worst enemy of your skin. Here is what sun does:

- Wrinkles the skin
- Darkens the skin, which makes folds stand out
- Creates age spots, moles and cancer
- Increases sagging of the skin (poor nutrition and a sluggish thyroid contribute)

Smoking is the second-worst wrinkle maker because it hampers blood flow to nourish the skin. Quitting smoking will reverse some of that damage. Skin renews itself often, and people on healthful diets have less wrinkles—no kidding. Make sure that the new building blocks are not pizza and donuts, but healthful, nutritious foods. (For more tips about your skin, see "Wrinkles" in chapter 14.)

PERSONAL HYGIENE

- **Care for your teeth or your dentures—your smile depends on them.** Brush and floss every day. Avoid sugars of all kind because they lead to gum disease. The healthiest tooth will fall out if your gums are chronically inflamed. Avoid toothpastes with coloring because they might worsen gum disease. Use a mouth rinse—a drop of tea tree oil or myrrh works well without harsh chemicals. Unsavory mouth bacteria are linked to heart disease and stroke, and bacteria from the mouth can start pneumonia in the elderly.

- **Use eyeglasses if you need them.** Squinting will only give you crow's feet—and not the kind that comes from laughter. Wrong glasses can lead to headaches and falls, so visit an eye doctor yearly. But for simple reading glasses, the cheap ones from the drug store are just fine. Sunglasses not only prevent wrinkles, they also protect your eyes from sun damage that leads to cataracts.

- **Pay attention to your hearing.** Do people have to repeat often what they have just said to you? Get an evaluation with an audiogram early. And if the doctor prescribes a hearing aid, WEAR IT! When you have bad eyes, you put on better glasses, and the problem is solved. No such luck with hearing aids. When you try out a hearing aid for the first time, you will experience confusion, anger and frustration. All the noises will be amplified—even those that you don't want to hear. It takes getting used to and is especially difficult in the company of many people. Start with wearing your hearing aid every day for ten minutes only, and slowly increase the time. Don't put it off "until it is really necessary," because then it might be too late, and you might never learn to use it. Hearing is important: Studies show that deaf and hard-of-hearing people are unhappier than blind people because they are missing out on all-important conversation. They become suspicious, jealous and lonely. So don't let the lifeline to a happier life lie around unused in a drawer!

- **Don't confuse sun and light.** Direct sun is harsh; light is healing and life-promoting. I advise everyone to take off their clothes at least once a day and expose every nook and cranny of their body to natural light. You can do this in the privacy of your home in a bedroom flooded with natural light, or even outdoors if you have a private, shaded deck. Light fights depression, vitamin D deficiency, cancer and skin diseases (especially fungal infections).

- **Stay clean.** Taking a daily shower or sponge bath boosts your mood, gets rid of bacteria and lets you face the world with confidence. I have seen patients who neglect themselves because they feel old and lonely. Unfortunately, neglecting your body will make you old and lonely.

Your Home Is Your Castle

Make your home your safe haven from where you venture out into the world. Your home should be filled with the colors and objects that give you pleasure.

- A bedroom that is clean, airy, quiet and dark.
- A simple kitchen where it is fun to cook, with a big pan (aluminum or coated cookware are

not recommended!), a pot, a couple of sharp knives, a metal spatula.

- A corner for quiet meditation and yoga. Some people keep special or meaningful objects here: religious symbols, candles, photographs of loved ones or beautiful places, shells or rocks collected on their travels, incense, even small, electric water fountains—whatever nourishes your soul.

- A place for your favorite books and activities—quilt making or woodworking or playing the banjo.

- A place, even if it is just your kitchen table, where you can sit with a friend and have a cup of tea or share a meal.

Protect Your Body—What to Avoid

If you fall off a cliff, you will not make it to 100, so avoid what can *really* hurt you:

- **Don't smoke.** Every time I see somebody smoking, it breaks my heart. My mother died of lung cancer at sixty-seven—way too early to go. Get help with smoking cessation. (See "Smoking" in chapter 14 for my suggestions of how to do this.) You might not break the habit on the first try, but one day you will. And from that day on, healing can start. Your kisses will taste fresher three days after quitting.

- **Don't drink alcohol in excess.** A glass of wine or beer a day (women have far smaller livers, so I recommend only half a glass) has health benefits, resulting in less heart disease and stroke. But drunkenness damages relationships as well as health. There is no excuse; get help if you cannot quit by yourself. In my experience as a doctor, alcoholism is often linked to food allergies, food intolerances, and a diet high in sugar and white starches.

- **Avoid direct sun.** It ages your skin and carries the risk of skin cancer. Check your body: The areas that usually are covered by clothes are probably still wrinkle-free. Most of the sun's harm, of course, has already been done before you reach drinking age. That makes it even more important to protect your skin now from further damage. Remember "slip, slap, slop": Slip on long-sleeved clothes, slap on a hat, slop on the sunscreen. A hat (or an umbrella) protects your scalp and the delicate skin of your face, neck and ears, all of which are favorite locations of skin cancer. For sun block, titanium-based is the best, but also the most expensive. Avoid sunburns. And forget about tanning and tanning booths. Did you know that nutrition high in antioxidants (vegetables and fruit) provides you with inside protection from sun damage?

- **Don't use coated or aluminum cookware.** Aluminum has been linked to Alzheimer's disease and dementia, and coating has become an environmental hazard.
- **Don't microwave your food as it destroys essential nutrients.** I don't even use a microwave for heating water.
- **Keep away from pesticides and herbicides.** Make sure your food and cosmetics are pesticide-free. Don't use herbicides in your garden. Learn about alternative ways. You only have to look at it from the window of an airplane to realize that our world, the "blue planet," has become very small, and there is no room anymore to hide the bad stuff. It will come back to haunt you (and your children and grandchildren) one day.
- **Avoid genetically manipulated food.** We don't know yet what they are doing to humans, but studies have shown that they are killing some

species like the monarch butterfly.

- **Don't overuse caffeine.** Caffeine is a nice stimulant, but people overdo it. A cup or two of coffee in the morning, an aromatic tea in the afternoon, are nice. But excess, again, is harmful. If you are hooked on caffeine, cut down only by one cup per week. If you cut down faster, you risk withdrawal headaches.

- **Curb unnecessary pharmaceuticals.** I rarely give a pill to a patient and then say: "You have to take this for the rest of your life." Instead, I make a plan with the patient to create a better lifestyle and work on slowly tapering the medication, under supervision, of course. Tell your physician that you want to become healthier and might be able to eliminate or decrease your medications after a few months. Make her your partner in this process.

- **Don't miss your regular checkups.** Get yearly PAP tests, prostate exams, eye exams, blood pressure checks and diabetic exams. Have a colonoscopy at fifty. Those should be the minimum. Mammograms and yearly flu shots are being hotly debated—but they have probable advantages. You should definitely have a tetanus shot every ten years—remember the date because your doctor likely will not. And once or twice in your lifetime you should have a pneumococcal vaccination—talk with your physician. When you travel abroad, get your shots and take the recommended medication.

HEALTHY TO 100 TIP

Buy long-term care (LTC) insurance before you are sixty. Find out if you are eligible for LTC insurance through your spouse or your work. This is what you need:

- An insurance firm that has been in business at least a dozen years (so that you know it is viable).
- Coverage for at least five years, affordable into your mid-eighties (that is when most people go into a nursing home).
- No grace period (zero elimination days), because otherwise you and your family may go broke before the insurance takes effect—you need it when you need it and not months later.
- Home health care coverage (because health insurance does not usually cover that).
- Inflation protection (so that it will actually cover the costs).

8

NOURISH YOUR BODY

*Let your food be your medicine, and
your medicine be your food.*

—Hippocrates (470–410 BC)

On your journey into aging, food can be your fuel or your heavy baggage—you decide.

Have you been looking for the perfect diet your whole life? Despite the claims of the fad diet books, the perfect diet does not exist. As our bodies are all different, so are our nutritional requirements. But you can discover *your* perfect diet simply by listening to your body.

Your body actually "tells" you what it needs. Aches and pains are the language of your body.

Heartburn? The tomatoes or fried chicken did not agree with you. Bloated? You ate too much or the wrong food. Stiff all over? Maybe you have a sensitivity to wheat. Bursitis? Try cutting out dairy. Headaches? Too much booze or coffee. Back pain? Are there cashews in your granola?

These, of course, are just examples. But what do we usually do when we experience discomfort? We reach for a pill. How many years did I take a pharmaceutical to soothe my esophagus on fire before I figured out that tomatoes triggered the pain? Let me give you some guidance on your way to better understanding your body and its needs.

Freshness

Freshness is the main "ingredient" in healthful foods. Health does not come from a vitamin bottle, a "slim" shake or a nutritional bar—our bodies have been nourished for many, many generations on the fresh things Mother Earth provides for us. Because of the freshness, it is better to eat an apple than an apple pie or apple juice. Worst of all is eating a cereal or a bar with "apple flavor."

Don't restrict the amount of fresh produce in your diet. You can have as much fruit and vegetables (cooked and raw) as you want. Just beware—the danger might lie in dressings, sauces and condiments.

Here are a few of the cancer-fighting compounds in vegetables and fruit (and there are hundreds or more!):

- Sulforaphane (broccoli and cabbages)
- Lycopene (tomatoes)
- Sinigrin (Brussels sprouts, horseradish, mustards)
- Beta carotene (apricots, broccoli, butternut squash, cantaloupe, carrots, kale, mustard greens, peaches, pumpkin, spinach, sweet potatoes)
- Carotenoids (in almost all fruit and vegetables)
- Lutein (asparagus, broccoli, brussels sprouts, collard greens, corn, kale, peas, Romaine lettuce, spinach, zucchini)

All these compounds are extremely bitter. Plants developed them because they ward off predators like insects and animals. That is why many of us often don't like veggies. But bitter is good for digestion—keep that in mind. And why not make your vegetables more palatable with olive oil, garlic, onions (they give a pleasant, sweet taste to any dish), and fresh or dried herbs? Besides, herbs will add more of the cancer-fighting compounds.

HEALTHY TO 100 TIP

Two good rules of thumb:

- Don't eat anything that contains ingredients on the label that you cannot pronounce. (Just try to read the label on a "diet" drink.)
- Don't buy anything for which you see an advertisement on television. They don't advertise an apple or a carrot.

Healthful Vegetable Soup

In a pot, glaze an onion in a teaspoon of olive oil. Add a cup of water. Rummage in your pantry for some dried herbs or spices and sprinkle them in generously. Add whatever vegetables you have at hand: a stalk of celery, two carrots, green beans, a chopped-up piece of cabbage, a few button mushrooms.

Add pepper and salt sparingly.

Bring to a boil, then simmer until still crisp— about five minutes.

This recipe serves one person, is easy to make— and it is different every time because of different vegetables, herbs and spices. You will never tire of it. You can also add meat, eggs, fish or shrimp for more protein, but it is already a satisfying meal in itself.

Healthful Vegetable Stir-Fry

You can use the Healthful Vegetable Soup recipe for a stir-fry—just add one to two tablespoons of olive oil and eliminate the water. Serve this with a whole grain, such as brown rice or quinoa, or a legume like split peas. My husband and I recently began to eat this stir-fry almost every night. It melted away the few pounds he had accumulated on his belly without any effort or deprivation.

Foods That Harm

Soft Drinks and Juices

Health-wise, you do not get your money back when you invest in soda drinks and juices. Buy fresh fruit and vegetables instead. Drink water: It is cheap (filtered water is cheaper than bottled water) and healthful; mankind has been drinking water since the dawn of history.

Sugar

It is not so much the sugar itself that hurts your health (glucose is one of the most important molecules in your body); it is the sheer amount of sugar (every year in the United States far more than 100 pounds of sugar is consumed per person) and the many ways sugar is hidden in our food. It is also the kind of sugar: Nutritionists are especially wary of high fructose corn syrup. But *no* sugar is healthful in large quantities.

By law, ingredients in food have to be labeled in the order of their decreasing weight in the food. To disguise the fact that sugar is often the first ingredient, manufacturers cleverly use different kinds of sugar in one product. These are all different names of sugars: high-fructose corn syrup, malt, barley malt, dextrose, fructose, honey, maple syrup, lactose, dextrose, corn syrup, brown sugar, molasses, cane sugar. Also avoid the sugar alcohols: isomalt, lactitol, mannitol, sorbitol, xylitol.

Do you know how much sugar is hidden in processed food? Here are some examples:

- 1 teaspoon of sugar in a tablespoon of tomato ketchup
- 10 teaspoons of sugar in a low-fat fruit yogurt

- 13 teaspoons of sugar in a 12-ounce can of soda
- 5 teaspoons of sugar in a small container of applesauce
- 5 teaspoons of sugar in a health bar advertised for slimming down
- Up to 1 teaspoon of sugar per hot dog
- 1 teaspoon of sugar per nutritional bar for diabetics (This last one I find especially outrageous as a doctor: Manufacturers are allowed to label something a *diabetic* food that has sugar in it! And patients eat it, thinking *the more the better* for their diabetes.)

Do not switch to artificial sweeteners. The jury is still out about their health dangers. Moreover, they never let you lose your sweet tooth. Because sugar causes food cravings, it is best to go "cold turkey" on the sugar you put in your food and your drinks and to avoid processed food with hidden sugars altogether.

Stevia is a sweet plant, available in health-food stores. You can try it in small amounts—but again, it will only feed your sweet tooth. Beet sugar and cane sugar are better than corn sugar—but only in very small amounts.

White Starches

Starches are nothing more than one molecule of sugar after the other, like beads strung onto a long string. Your saliva, when you chew, clips those sugar molecules from the chain. In effect, white starches are no better than sugar. Avoid:

- Baked goods and bread made from white flour
- Cornstarch
- Potato starch
- Potatoes and sweet potatoes. They are rather high in starches and should be eaten sparingly—definitely not daily.

Fried Foods and Hydrogenated Fats

These fats promote cancer and inflammation in your body and should be eliminated without regret. Besides, fried food is loaded with calories.

Dairy

We have been inundated with misleading advertising about healthful milk and milk products. After a certain age (about when you enter kindergarten), you definitely don't need milk anymore. Let me give you the many reasons:

- Milk is a high-caloric liquid that is contributing heavily (pun intended) to our present epidemic of overweight, which comprises more than 60 percent of the adult population. When I grew up in Europe after World War II, children were starving, and milk was a godsend for them. In our affluent society, milk is hazardous.

- Dairy adds more protein to our already too protein-rich fare. The extra protein is digested and broken down to acidic purines, which need buffering before they can be expelled from the body. Your body takes the alkaline calcium from your bones to buffer the acidic purines, thus promoting bone loss.

- Dairy is a mucus-producing food, bad for asthma, bronchitis and hay fever.

- Dairy promotes inflammation in your body, thus creating or exacerbating arthritis, bursitis, tendonitis, heart disease, diabetes and cancer (among others).

- Milk and milk products may contain residuals from pesticides, hormones and antibiotics, all of which increase your risk of cancer.

- Many people (especially Asians and African-Americans, but many Caucasians, too) are lactose intolerant and suffer from heartburn and indigestion without knowing the cause.

If you think you cannot live without cheese and yogurt, you might be allergic to dairy. Cravings are one of the signs of allergies and food intolerances. Cows don't drink milk (calves do). Cows eat grass—and have very strong bones. Cows have, admittedly, a different stomach from us, but I am not asking you to eat grass. Just stick to green, leafy vegetables such as kale, dandelion greens, lettuces and broccoli. (Go easy on Swiss chard and spinach, which are high in oxalates.) Herbs are also a good source of calcium. Indeed, most vegetables contain calcium—and in a form that is more easily absorbed than the calcium from dairy or from pills.

If you had a cow in your backyard and drank your own milk and made your own yogurt and cheese, I would not be quite as stern about dairy. But what we buy in the supermarket is a far cry from the original product directly from the udder. Even the organic milk now has an expiration date a month away—clearly, not an unadulterated food.

Good milk would turn into sour milk within a day or two.

Don't get desperate about what you can't eat after all these no-nos. Try, for instance, not to eat milk, cheese and yogurt for a week. Observe how you feel. Then splurge on a cheese pizza—and again, just observe, don't judge. How does your stomach feel? Are heartburn, migraines, joint pains, cravings returning? Do you feel exhausted, tired, depressed? After a while, you will understand your body's needs. For some people, dairy is like poison. Others (few indeed) might get away with it. It depends on your genes and ancestry. See the sidebar "High-Calcium Foods" on page 71 for nondairy foods that are high in calcium.

Foods That Heal

Vegetables

Choose vegetables that are colorful because the colors are powerful antioxidants, furthering longevity and helping to fight cancer (among other diseases). Most vegetables should be cooked, but a daily salad is in order. Cooking predigests the food and makes many nutrients better available. Just don't overcook because then you lose the vitamins. Cook to a crunch—that is the best. Steaming is the most healthful method, but I have to admit that I also find it the most boring. It turns out that adding some fat—preferably olive oil— will help your body use the fat-dependant vitamins A, D, E and K. I mostly panfry my vegetables with olive oil at not too high heat.

Some people, especially if not originating from South America, have difficulties with the night- shade family (eggplant, peppers [except black], potatoes, tomatoes). Observe yourself. Perhaps tomatoes have given you that heartburn for many years.

With vegetables, be adventurous beyond iceberg lettuce and broccoli: Try rutabaga, turnips and beets, green beans, peas, cucumbers, summer and winter squashes, all kinds of cabbages, burdock roots, parsnips. Go to an ethnic market and dis- cover vegetable varieties that are new to you and inexpensive.

Mushrooms

Mushrooms (button, chanterelles, maitake, morels, oyster, porcini, portabella, reishi, shiitake, truffles) boost your immune system, but fresh mushrooms are rather expensive. I buy cut and dried mushrooms at the Chinese market for pennies. My favorites are auricularia and white fungus (tremella). All I have to do is steep them in hot water for a moment, then add them to my stir-fry. The cooled water I use on my flowers. Never eat uncooked mushrooms; they are toxic.

Fruit

What do you think are more healthful—fruit or vegetables? No, it's not fruit! We have been so trained about how important fruits are that we now often take them as a quick veggie substitute. No peeling and chopping, no cooking. Fruit should be reserved for dessert and the snack in-between meals.

Having put in a word for vegetables, I must admit that fruit is loaded with healthful vitamins (especially A and C) and antioxidants. Just go a little light on tropical fruit if your family tree does not stem from the tropics. And listen to your body. Some people overeat fruit, and some people cannot stomach acidic fruit like oranges. And remember: Orange juice is not a fruit! Stick to the *whole* fruit.

FOODS HIGHEST IN VITAMIN C

The fruits highest in vitamin C are not common fare here: Acerola and camu camu both have vitamin C contents ranging in the thousands of milligrams. Compare that with a meager 6 milligrams in an apple. Only rosehips come close, with 1,500 milligrams, but you have to cook them and add sugar before they are palatable. The following are other fruits that are good sources of vitamin C:

- Berries
- Cantaloupe
- Grapefruit
- Guava
- Kiwi
- Orange
- Papaya
- Pineapple
- Strawberries (commercial strawberries are loaded with pesticides—only organic ones are recommended)

And don't forget vegetables: Broccoli, cauliflower (all cabbages, actually), green peppers, leafy greens (chards, collards, dandelion greens, dinosaur kale, kale, mustard greens, red beet greens, turnip greens, and so on) and tomatoes are high in vitamin C, too. So is grass-fed meat. Surprise, surprise!

HIGH-CALCIUM FOODS (NONDAIRY)

These are good options for getting the calcium you need while avoiding dairy:

- All greens, including herbs
- Cabbage
- Cauliflower
- Celery
- Dulse
- Irish moss
- Kelp
- Lemons
- Nuts and seeds

Fish and Seafood

Fish would be perfect fare if not for the mercury pollution (among other pollutants) that now renders especially large fish like albacore tuna, king mackerel, shark, swordfish and tilefish rather unhealthful. So don't eat them more often than once a month. But smaller fish are safe twice a week—even for children and pregnant women: catfish, pollock, sardines, wild salmon. Shrimp are fine, too. They are high in vitamin D. Freshwater fish do not have the amount of healthful omega-3s that seawater fish have, but they are still a good source of protein. Because of diseases in freshwater fish, they need to be thoroughly cooked before serving.

Meats, Poultry and Game

These should be eaten sparingly; aim for not more than twice a week and in very moderate amounts. Safe rule of thumb: cut your portions in half (saves money, too!). The problem with our meats is that the animals are grain-fed, which is unnatural. It makes for unhealthy animals with unhealthy guts. Then they are given hormones and antibiotics and are exposed to pesticides and other pollutants—unless you buy organic (which I recommend if you can afford it).

HEALTHY TO 100 TIP

Eat lamb. Lambs are born, thrown out on the pasture and then harvested without ever getting grain-fed or given hormones. Unfortunately, lamb is expensive and quite fatty. Cut off the visible fat and enjoy it in small amounts.

Vegetarian Dishes

If you have fish and meat each twice a week, that leaves three days without either. On those days, try tofu, tempeh or mushrooms. All these also provide proteins, as do whole grains, legumes and nuts. Only people who work hard physically need higher amounts of protein.

Nuts, Seeds and Nut Butters

Nuts and seeds are another protein source—if you are not allergic to them. Sprinkle them over cereal or vegetables, or eat them as a meal together with a fruit. Nuts have quite a few calories but healthful fats. Of course, if you have three meals a day and then snack on nuts, they will only bolster your "love handles." But if you substitute a meal with nuts, you benefit from their bounty of vitamins, minerals and omega-3 fatty acids (the fat your body needs).

Herbs, Spices and Seaweed

All herbs are plants, so you think they are no different from fruit and vegetables, right? But they are. Herbs are much stronger and loaded with more nutrients than even vegetables: vitamins, minerals (especially calcium!), antioxidants, and so on. (Pregnant women and babies should use them cautiously or not at all.) But sprinkle them daily and deliberately over your food.

Make use of *all* the plant world, and spice up your meals with healthful herbs and spices:

Allspice	Curry
Anise	Dill
Arugula	Fennel
Basil	Fenugreek
Bay leaves	Garlic
Black pepper	Ginger
Capers	Horseradish
Caraway	Hyssop
Cardamom	Juniper berries
Celery seeds	Lemon balm
Chervil	Lemon grass
Chili (nightshades!)	Lovage
Chives	Mace
Cilantro	Marjoram
Cinnamon	Mints
Clove	Nutmeg
Coriander	Onion (*I view it as both*
Cumin	*a vegetable and a spice.*)

READER/CUSTOMER CARE SURVEY

We care about your opinions! Please take a moment to fill out our online Reader Survey at
http://survey.hcibooks.com. As a **"THANK YOU"** you will receive a **VALUABLE INSTANT COUPON** towards future
book purchases as well as a **SPECIAL GIFT** available only online! Or, you may mail this card back to us
and we will send you a copy of our exciting catalog with your valuable coupon inside.

First Name _____ MI. _____ Last Name _____

Address _____ City _____

State _____ Zip _____ Email _____

1. Gender	**4. Annual**	**6. Marital Status**
❑ Female ❑ Male	**Household Income**	❑ Single
	❑ under $25,000	❑ Married
2. Age	❑ $25,000 - $34,999	❑ Divorced
❑ 8 or younger	❑ $35,000 - $49,999	❑ Widowed
❑ 9-12 ❑ 13-16	❑ $50,000 - $74,999	
❑ 17-20 ❑ 21-30	❑ over $75,000	**Comments**
❑ 31+		
	5. What are the	
3. Did you receive	**ages of the children**	
this book as a gift?	**living in your house?**	
❑ Yes ❑ No	❑ 0 - 14 ❑ 15+	

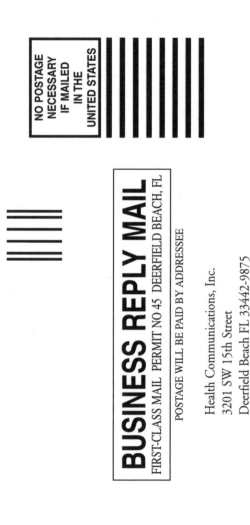

BUSINESS REPLY MAIL

FIRST-CLASS MAIL PERMIT NO 45 DEERFIELD BEACH, FL

POSTAGE WILL BE PAID BY ADDRESSEE

Health Communications, Inc.

3201 SW 15th Street

Deerfield Beach FL 33442-9875

Orange peel

Oregano

Paprika and cayenne
peppers *(but be aware
that these two are night-
shades that could make
joint pains, etc., worse—
observe yourself)*

Poppy seeds

Rosemary

Sacred basil

Saffron

Sage

Savory

Scallion

Tarragon

Thyme

Turmeric

Vanilla

Verbena

Wasabi

Watercress

What a list! And each plant offers you its healthful, healing molecules, not to mention worlds of
taste and flavor!

How many of these have you ever used in cooking? I sprinkle them in turns on pre-cooked and
heated up organic beans (from a can), and voilà! A
perfect fast food when I don't feel like cooking.

Seaweeds

Full of minerals, they are especially loaded
with healthful iodine. Use ground seaweeds in
your salads—they are made from kelp, nori and

dulse. Or eat a piece of dulse or nori (kelp tastes a bit boring) as a snack to fulfill your craving for something chewy. They are high in salt, however, so eat them regularly but sparingly. (Not for people whose thyroid has gone wild.)

Grains

These staples are cheap and versatile. Beside carbohydrates, they contain proteins (Teff, amaranth and quinoa are highest in protein.) Grains should be eaten whole. The recipe is easy: For most grains, cook one cup of grain to two cups of water with a pinch of salt. Once the water has boiled, turn heat on low, cover with a lid and let simmer until all fluid is gone. (The time will be different for each kind of grain.) Unusual grains to consider include:

- Amaranth
- Brown rice (comes in several forms, but basically long and short. Long cooks dry and aromatic, whereas short is sweet and sticky. I like especially the blackish-cooking dark brown rice.)
- Buckwheat
- Bulgur (wheat)

- Couscous (wheat)
- Kasha (a pre-roasted buckwheat)
- Millet
- Quinoa
- Teff
- Wheat berries
- Wild rice (not actually a rice and may cause problems for people with gluten intolerance)

Legumes

Legumes are beans, peas and garbanzos. My favorites are chana dal, split peas and European soldier beans. Try different ones and find out how your body reacts. Leftover grains and legumes are great for breakfast and in full-meal salads (with olive oil and lemon dressing, *not* mayonnaise; add a raw, chopped onion). I do not recommend corn because high-fructose corn syrup has been introduced in so many food items that people are getting more and more intolerant of corn. Listen to what your body tells you. All grains and legumes might be rendered more digestible by soaking, fermenting and/or roasting.

Fats and Oils

Fats are solid, oils are fluid—but biochemically, they are all fats. Without fats, you cannot survive. Our brain, for example, contains more than 90 percent fat. Each cell in our bodies is surrounded by a cell wall that is nearly pure fat. On the other hand, very low-fat diets (like the Ornish diet) have been proven to help heart patients—if they manage to stick with it, which is hard.

The discussion about fats is not yet closed. Animal fats (particularly from grass-fed animals) might not be the culprits for heart disease. But for the time being, as we have no better data yet, sticking to the olive oil-based Mediterranean diet is a good idea.

Chocolate

Chocolate is a healthful food—in moderation. What makes chocolate unhealthful (and makes people crave it in indecent amounts) are the milk and corn sugar with which cheap chocolates are adulterated. Find an organic dark chocolate (expensive but worthwhile) without milk and made with cane sugar, and have one tiny piece at a time. Melt it on your tongue and feel blessed.

An affordable alternative to satisfy your craving for chocolate is *sugarless* baker's chocolate, available in every supermarket. They come in handy cubes, wrapped in singles. They are so bitter that you will never be in danger of overeating. Lick one.

9

PAINLESS
WEIGHT LOSS

Are you wearing yourself out prematurely because you are carrying too much weight along on your journey through life? I have lost some prospective patients when they heard about my weight-loss program. I remember one woman rushing in, demanding to know: "I have to lose sixty pounds from now to September—to fit in my wedding gown. Will you help me?" It was May, and the answer was "No!"

My rules are easy—and never, ever involve hunger or abusing your body—but they do take time:

- **Everything that goes into your mouth should be fresh and unprocessed** (cooking allowed, of course!).
- **Stop all soft drinks immediately.** Drink filtered water and herbal tea instead.
- **Lose no more than two pounds per month—** but lose those pounds for good.
- **Add exercise to your day,** as little as a few minutes, because otherwise you lose muscle tissue with the fat tissue—which you don't want to do.
- **Celebrate every meal:** set the table nicely, even if you are alone; light a candle; play soothing music in the background; do not read or watch TV. Never eat while you are doing other things—like watching a movie, driving, and so on. Saying grace might help you.
- **No seconds.**
- **Don't snack mindlessly.** Always have some nuts, fruit or a tiny piece of dark chocolate for when you feel faint with hunger and the next meal is not in sight.
- **Don't eat while watching TV.** Exercise instead.
- **Don't munch at the movies.** You came for the entertainment, not to get fat.

- **Don't taste while cooking.** Amazingly, you can smell if salt or pepper or something is missing in the dish. Try it. A tablespoon that you nibble while cooking may have 100 calories in it. You could easily amass a second meal on your hips just by tasting before dinner has even started.
- **Learn why you eat for all the wrong reasons:** stress, boredom, greed, loneliness, and so on. Keep a food journal to figure out why and when you eat.
- **Learn about your natural body size.** Stop dreaming of that waiflike body if you come from a family of big-boned amazons. Knowing your BMI (body mass index) might help you. (Ask your doctor for your BMI or look it up on the Internet.) If you are big-boned, stay at the higher end of your range; stay at the lower end if you have delicate bones.
- **No diet pills, slimming drinks, weight-loss bars,** or whatever advertisements want to sell you.
- **Improve your bowel health** with an acidophilus preparation.
- **Don't keep *unhealthful* foods in your fridge or your pantry.**
- **Don't go shopping when you are hungry.**

- **Never try to stay on your diet at a grand celebration.** For that one special day, forget all the rules and eat what you want. The next day, write in your journal how it made you feel. Happy? Depressed? Bloated? Achy? Remorseful? Then get back on the wagon and continue your travel to a lighter, healthier you. (This does not apply to business meetings or every family birthday if you happen to have twenty-six grandchildren!)
- **Don't believe that a liquid diet, diet pills or fast programs can melt your fat away.** You will be left fat *and* poor! Not to mention flabby.

I am wary of too much weight loss in too short a time. So if you lose faster, you may gloat—but pay extra attention not to push it. And keep it up.

Think about this: If you lose only one pound, *one single pound*, you have already broken the cycle of continuous weight gain from high school to grave that seems so inevitable in our American culture. If you lose one pound and keep it off, you have not gained the twenty-five other pounds that were likely to accumulate.

And another thought: If you lose only five pounds, you have turned the metabolism of your body around and have started *healing*.

More Than Fat

Of course, fat on your body is a sign that you are taking in more calories than you are using up. But not everybody metabolizes food in the same way—some people really gain faster, especially after menopause. Life is not fair.

But you cannot lose weight successfully if you haven't taken the huge burden from your heart. I have seen again and again that overweight people not only carry the burden of their weight; they often carry an emotional burden as well. The German poet Johann Wolfgang von Goethe described it: "Mankind's whole misery weighs on my shoulders." Overweight people often feel that their suffering is a given. It is not. You just have to face what burdens you.

If you have had heartbreak in your past—a sad childhood, abuse, anger, a broken home, a big trauma—and you have not begun to work out those past hurts you will not get very far. First address the old hurts, then move on, eat better, exercise more. And give yourself slack: It will not be done overnight; it will be a lifelong struggle. Get help from a friend, a group, a therapist, and learn to deal with your pain.

Also know that food allergies or food intolerances can make you crave more of that food. Do you binge? Are you never able to stop after a few bites? Do you have to eat the whole package? Do you feel sorry and ashamed afterward? It's not *you* doing this—the food is making you do it. Learn to avoid the foods that trigger binging and cravings.

Specific Food Suggestions for Losing Weight

- **Fill yourself with healthful foods.** How many of these did you have this week? Avocados, onions, garbanzos, celery, prunes, olive oil, beans, black tea, green tea, herbal tea, organic eggs, fish, flaxseed, blueberries, lentils, spinach, tempeh, kale, celeriac, rutabaga, whole grains, almonds, artichokes, broccoli, cantaloupe, garlic, apples, carrots, raw nuts, turkey, Swiss chard, pumpkin. And this is just a tiny portion of earth's bounty!

  If you have this wide a variety of vegetables, fruit and nuts, you will never ever have to think again about *fiber*. Fiber is in all of them, naturally and abundantly.

SNACK IDEAS

- A few nuts—what can fit into a heaping tablespoon, not more.
- One tiny bit of dark chocolate (no milk; cane sugar only).
- A piece of fruit. Apples are among the most healthful. My favorite varieties are Braeburn, Gaia, Fuji.
- A piece of dulse or nori (seaweed).
- Raw vegetables (carrot, celery, jicama, cauliflower, to name a few).
- A piece of heavy, whole grain bread dipped in half a teaspoon of olive oil.
- A few olives.
- A can of sardines.
- _____
- _____
- _____
- _____

Copy this list and post it on your fridge. Add to it when you have found another healthful snack. These are *not* healthful: crackers, yogurt, cheese, Oreos, Slim Jim (or similar products).

Not all of these suggestions work for everybody. I found that I need some fat or protein; otherwise I will get ravenous. Since I developed an allergy to nuts, I now do well on dark chocolate, in tiny morsels.

HEALTHY TO 100 TIP

To visit a restaurant and not fall back into bad habits:

- Choose a restaurant that has reasonable fare. A fast-food outlet, for instance, will have nothing "healthful" but an overpriced, limp salad.
- Drink water—without ice.
- Focus on vegetables and salads.
- A baked potato is not a bad choice if you avoid toppings like sour cream and butter. Don't try mashed potatoes; they likely come from a package.
- Go easy on bread and butter.
- Avoid everything "fried," "breaded" or "stuffed."
- Avoid cheese, cream and sausage.
- Choose healthful entrees like baked or broiled fish.
- Eat lamb, but remove the visible fat, and eat a small portion only. Nobody needs to down six lamb cutlets. Take the rest home in a doggie bag.
- Ask for a no-cheese, vegetables-only pizza.
- Spaghetti with tomato sauce and a salad is not so bad, but Seafood Alfredo is.

10

WHY EXERCISE?

Your journey into the prime of life and beyond will not be accomplished sitting around. You will have to *walk* there. We are animals made for roaming the savanna. Our bodies and metabolism depend on exercise—not to mention our mood and happiness.

If you are not into exercise, don't be discouraged. Centenarians did not get to the ripe old age of 100 by doing aerobic exercise at the gym. They did it by keeping busy. They also, of course, started their lives when much more manual labor was common. So we have to make up for all the advantages of washing machines, cars and vacuum cleaners, with a little effort.

Here is the pep talk I give my patients: Exercise not only helps your muscles, heart, blood pressure, metabolic state, lung function and weight loss, but it also improves all aspects of brain function such as: mood and memory, and it may even help prevent Alzheimer's disease. Exercise:

- Is the key to feeling younger and more energetic.
- Makes you look younger.
- Brings blood to your brain, heart and muscles.
- Decreases depression and anxiety.
- Strengthens your heart.
- Increases your metabolic rate and makes you burn calories faster.
- Builds up muscles, which in turn *help you lose weight in your sleep*.
- Keeps your joints flexible.
- Elevates HDL, the *good* cholesterol.
- Prevents falls and their dreaded complications of hip fractures and pneumonia.
- Produces sweat, which detoxifies your body.
- Helps diabetes (by lowering insulin resistance), high and low blood pressure, and a host of other illnesses.
- Improves breathing capacity.
- Strengthens the immune system and helps

prevent infections and cancer.
- Improves your sleep.
- Reduces swelling in your feet.

In fact, exercise is such an age-fighter, it is probably even more important than proper eating habits—if only for the reason that exercise seems to curb your appetite, whereas eating does not entice you to move more. You won't get far on your journey to the prime of your life without exercise.

Without exercise, physical decline is inevitable. You might think that your brain and your heart are the most important parts of your body, but what really ages people is the loss of muscle mass. And it is not age per se that does it; it is inactivity.

The most amazing thing about moving is that you are building up your muscles with everything you do. And then, in your sleep, these better muscles help you lose more weight because muscle has a higher metabolic rate than fat tissue. It is a built-in reward: You lose once while you exercise, and a second time while you sleep.

And every little bit helps. Studies on the very elderly (eighty-five-plus) showed that even exercise done in a chair (such as moving arms, legs and shoulders) has a positive impact on balance, mood and stamina. And the best news is, with exercise, you lower your chances of breaking a hip.

Nothing keeps you young like exercise. If you did everything else right, but weren't exercising— well, that's like cooking without water.

HEALTHY TO 100 TIP

Could you go for a ten-minute walk? Make it a habit—if possible, around noon every day, to take advantage of the sunlight. Or in a more southern climate, walk in the evening to walk the day's stress out of your system. Of course, you are allowed to walk longer than ten minutes—but ten is the minimum.

If for any health reason a walk around the block is not feasible, start with something easier. Studies have shown that at *any* age or *any* physical condition, you still improve with exercise. You are in a wheelchair? Lift your arms, holding two water bottles, and gently roll your neck.

How to Dodge "The Big Workout" and Still Get the Benefits of Exercise

If you are like me, you loathe the boredom of gyms and lengthy workout routines. But without exercise, there is only early death and a long road of suffering first. So these are the many little things I do during the day to dodge the big workout:

- Use stairs instead of elevators and escalators.
- Do knee lifts to strengthen my abdomen while waiting for the computer to download.
- Turn housecleaning into a fun workout with bends and stretches.
- Work in the garden.
- Use a bike for shopping instead of the car.
- Do a short yoga routine every day (mine lasts all of eleven minutes).
- Do ten pull-ups at a bar above the doorway whenever I pass it.
- Use a rowing machine (or any other home trainer) in front of the TV. I don't allow myself to watch a program without slowly working out—the entire length of the show.
- Hop on the spot whenever I have a few seconds to spare.
- Carry my own groceries—it's weight training and good for my spine.
- Periodically clean out the yard, attic and basement.
- Dance—from square dance to ballroom waltz, even just to the radio. And yes, my

husband and I still do a few turns of rock-and-roll.

- Do stretches or move up and down stairs and along the long corridor while on the phone.
- Have a ball handy; throw it to a wall and catch it. A minute a day will increase coordination and balance and will work on your arm flab. Play!
- Use two water-filled plastic bottles like dumbbells.
- Walk with a friend several times per week in a hilly neighborhood. I walk with my husband around the block after dinner every night. If it is raining, we don rubber boots and rain gear.

During exercise, always breathe through your nose and close your mouth, especially outside and in cold weather.

Of course, I never do *all of it* on any given day. It's just a menu I choose from. Every little bit helps. What are your obstacles to getting moving? For me it was the wrong self-image: "I am not athletic." You don't have to be an athlete to jump on the spot for a minute or stroll around the block. You just have to *do* it.

Fifty percent of Americans drop their exercise routines within half a year of starting them. I think it has to do with being overly ambitious. If you do two minutes on your treadmill or walk ten minutes around the block, pat yourself on the back and be proud of yourself. We cannot keep up huge exercise schedules; nobody can. So be light on yourself. And stick with it.

HEALTHY TO 100 TIP

For everyone in the second half of life, I particularly recommend the ancient Chinese practice of tai chi—a series of slow, flowing exercise movements originating from Traditional Chinese Medicine. Here is why: Major fractures due to falls are frequently fatal in older people. Studies have shown that the regular practice of tai chi improves balance, coordination and strength in the elderly and helps to prevent falls.

A 1996 study found that elderly people who took a tai chi course reduced their risk of falling by 47.5 percent compared with a control group that took a training course in balance.[32] Another study compared tai chi to balance training, strength training and combined balance and strength training in people with an average age of eighty. Those who learned tai chi gained significantly more balance and strength than the other groups.[33]

11

THE COLD IS
GOOD FOR YOU!

No life happens in good weather only. Nights are colder than days; seasons bring delightful sunshine but also rain and drizzle, ice and snow. Do you wish you were living in a place with the most perfect weather on Earth, like Hawaii? Well, wish again. You would be missing out on an important factor: healthful stress.

Mankind has always been exposed to the weather—and complained about it, no doubt. But research has shown that the cold can jumpstart a sluggish immune system and bring the complicated metabolism of people into higher gear.

Fresh air, cold water, ice and snow, rain and shine are there for free to stimulate your body into perfect health. Instead of shunning the cold, seek it! Bundle up and go for a short walk. Rain moisturizes your skin, and you air out your lungs. The nippy breeze makes you not only *feel* alive—it *keeps* you alive. You know that you will return to your snug home and can change into dry clothes.

Talking about snug, never keep the thermostat higher than 70 degrees F. Wear long pants and a sweater at home. Too much comfort lulls your immune system into laziness.

A trick to harvest the cold: Use cold water whenever feasible. Wash your hands with cold water, let the water run over your arms, walk barefoot at the beach and let the waves break over your feet. Take a very cold shower after every hot shower (discuss this with your physician if you have uncontrolled high blood pressure, heart disease or narrowing of your arteries). Research shows that cold water exposure on your skin improves your immune system and helps fight colds and cancer.[34]

Worried about air pollution? The truth is, except for very rare occasions (and they are usually announced over the radio and TV), indoor pollution is much worse. Open your window as often as possible to aerate your home. The best idea is to sleep with your window open. The trick is to have plenty of covers and use a shawl over your head. You can prewarm your bed with an electric heater—but I would not use it when you are in the bed.

12

BREATHING

God breathed life into Adam. Without breath, there is no life. Most of the time, we are not aware of our breath. It is automatic. Some people are naturally great breathers. (They usually are athletic and physically active.) Some are not. How often do I have to tell patients that their breathing is shallow? Most often it is not due to a disease. But in the long run, you snuff out your life force earlier if you are not breathing right.

A yoga class is a good way to start learning about breath. The yoga technique called "pranayama" is all about increasing your life force through deep, full breathing. Try it now. Breathe out, then take in a breath through your nose slowly and keep inhaling until you fill your entire chest and abdomen. No holding, just exhale slowly. How did that feel? Think of all the life-giving oxygen you have just brought into your body, and all of the toxic air you expelled. Take a few of these breaths when you are upset or exhausted.

Living with a Disability: A Portrait of Elinor

When Elinor had a stroke at seventy-three that incapacitated her right arm and leg, she was sure that she would never do anything useful again. From the time she was a child, her mother had taught her knitting, crocheting, sewing and other crafts, and she had become proficient in each. "I was really down and depressed after the stroke," she says. "After spending time in a rehabilitation hospital and having occupational and physical therapy, I could take care of myself and walk with a cane, but I was awkward and clumsy. My writing was terrible, and I had given up hope of ever doing the handicraft work I loved."

Then she and her husband moved into an independent living apartment at a senior residence. There, she signed up for a yoga class. "The breathing exercises helped me feel more in control," she says. "Shortly after we arrived, some of the women asked if I would join their knitting club," remembers Elinor. The group had been started about a year before and had come up with the idea of making blankets for the young teens in a homeless shelter. "Our mottos were *Knitting with a Purpose* and *Never Too Old to Care*," says Mimi, the group's founder and leader. An energetic woman of eighty-three, Mimi is a former social worker known both for her creative ideas and her ability to make things happen.

Elinor was initially reluctant to join the knitting group, but decided to try one meeting. "I went that first time with a ho-hum attitude," she remembers. "I wanted to please my new friends, but expected nothing for myself. I was sure that my knitting days were over. They gave me some needles and yarn, and I fiddled around for about ten minutes. Then my hand got tired, so I had a cup of tea and went home. That was all I felt good for."

Her friends encouraged her to try again, and she soon found herself there every week, sitting in a circle with the others, knitting as best she could and chatting. "Everyone was sweet and encouraging, tea time was fun, and I enjoyed being with them, so I kept it up," she says. The women were knitting large squares of yarn in bright colors.

When they had enough for a blanket, they would spread the squares on the floor and decide together on the arrangement. "Simplicity is key," says Mimi. "We all use the same size needles, the same number of stitches, and knit the same size squares. Then we all have a say in how the squares are put together. We insist that each blanket be beautiful and in good taste, the best we can turn out. Creating something for children who are homeless and poor means that we try harder!"

Within a few weeks, Elinor's knitting speed and stamina had improved, and she began taking needles and yarn back to her apartment to keep working. "Somewhere along the line, I realized that I was producing as many squares as anyone else," she says. "I wasn't even aware of it happening, but with their encouragement, I went from feeling helpless and useless to saying, 'Hey, I can do this!' I began to notice that my right hand was growing stronger and more agile in other ways as well. I could write and do small motor tasks more easily."

Under Mimi's leadership, the knitting club has grown from three to more than twenty committed women. "The group gives us the chance to socialize while contributing to our community," says Mimi. "Knitting is excellent physical therapy for old hands, and helping others with purposeful activity alleviates or even prevents the depression that is common to older people." (Knitting has, in fact, been called "the new Yoga," and is being touted as an excellent stress-reduction method.)

Within just a few months, Elinor had regained all of her former knitting prowess. "I became one of the knitting consultants and blanket finishers, crocheting together the completed squares," she says. But she didn't stop there. "The shelter staff told us that they also needed scarves for the kids as well as slippers for them to wear in the centers after they leave their snowy or muddy shoes in the hallway. And the teenage moms needed sweaters and baby clothes for their children." Working with Mimi, Elinor designed a simple way to make slippers out of leftover yarn. They also designed a child-sized sweater made out of extra blanket squares. "Nothing goes to waste," says Elinor.

"We've got some absolutely gorgeous blanket designs coming up," says Mimi. "Being in our eighties and nineties (with a few seventies) doesn't faze us. In fact, we hope we will encourage other groups in the community to get involved in keeping our children warm and letting them know we care."

13

HERBS AND
PHARMACEUTICALS

When I entered an American drugstore for the first time in my life, I saw an aspirin bottle that contained 1,000 pills. Then I found bottles just as large for Tylenol and ibuprofen. In Germany, aspirin was usually sold in glass tubes of 10 to 20 pieces (at least it was then). It struck me how different the cultures must be. In Germany, when you get a headache, you try to figure out why you got it: Overeating? Overdrinking? Bad boss? Nagging spouse? The weather? (Europeans have a way of blaming the weather for a lot of things.) Lack of exercise? Too much exercise? You get the idea.

Americans are more pragmatic. All they want is for the pain to go away. To that end, many pop pills. By the handful. But ibuprofen and the whole group of painkillers we call nonsteroidals can give you high blood pressure, bleeding from your intestines, kidney and liver failure. You can end up in dialysis, as many chronic pill gobblers have discovered. It is unlikely that it will happen after one or two pills, but after 1,000?

Not only are Americans pill happy, but their doctors are, too. Somehow, doctors think they haven't done their job if you leave the office without a prescription in your hand. And they add up. A senior citizen takes on average more than thirty prescription drugs per year. Let's not talk about health care cost. Let's just mention the side effects. As a board-certified internist, I cannot remember all the side effects of a single drug or the interactions between two drugs—let alone thirty! It seems the more drugs we get from physicians, the less time they have to really listen to our complaints.

Don't get me wrong. You have to take drugs for some diseases. But ailments that are caused by lifestyle, including stress, can be effectively treated without drugs. One way is through medicinal herbs.

I do not advocate taking herbs like pills, but herbs at least are not alien molecules that your body has difficulty recognizing and metabolizing. Herbs have been with us always. Herbs are nature's pharmacy. Use them—but use them in moderation.

My hero in herbs is botanist James A. Duke, Ph.D., the author of *The Green Pharmacy* and about forty other books about medicinal plants for health. I have taken several herbal and botanical courses with him, and whenever I am turning to a new health topic that interests me, I can be sure that he has been there before me—fifteen to twenty years earlier. His knowledge and breadth of interest is amazing. Amazing like the Amazon— Jim is an expert on, among many other things, medicinal plants of the Amazonian rainforest.

At one of his herb courses, I heard a young woman say about him: "Wow! I didn't know that a man of seventy-four could be that sexy!" I hope that young lady will one day find out that not everything is over after age thirty. "Sexy" wouldn't have been the first adjective I would have chosen to describe Jim Duke, but "alive," "interesting" and "vigorous" come to my mind. But what else does "sexy" mean if not a powerful life force reaching out?

If you were on a field trip with Jim Duke, you

would see him putting things into his mouth all the time—he calls it "harvesting from the wild." Once in a while, I'd frown when he'd do this because I'd consider the berry or leaf poisonous. "Keeps me alive," Jim laughs, "and I only eat tiny amounts." (Don't try this yourself. None of us has the knowledge that he has.)

I don't think it is by coincidence that Jim Duke is as vigorous and alive at his age as he is. Plants are his life's passion, and such passions and curiosity are what keep us alive. But then I wouldn't dismiss the herbs he is constantly ingesting. He is feeding his brain, his heart, all his organs the right food— natural plants.

Jim Duke's Healing Herbs

In addition to plants, Jim Duke loves music and has composed several songs. One of them is below, a parody of *Pistol* ("pistil") *Packing Momma*:

The only herb I take; On every single day
Cel'ry lowers uric acid; And keeps the gout away.
The drug it costs a whole lot more; The allopurinol
Cel'ry does it just as well, It really works, you all.
Feel them coming on, Bronchitis, colds and flus?
I'll take echinacea; The herb I always choose.

I also take the garlic, almost every day

The grandkids kinda shy away, AND keeps their germs away

I often memorize my lines; But sometimes I do not

That's when I take my ginkgo; But, YOU GOT IT, I forgot

Bilberries, blueberries, craisins, and grapes, the vine called
     Vitis

That's where we get the raisins, To master maculitis

Travel is bedraggling; Airports such a mess!

That's when I take my kava, To mellow down the stress

Zoloft is more often used, But old Saint John is best

Puts you in a better mood, With fewer side effects.

Prostate glands will grow; When old age comes along

When I take saw palmetto; Don't tinkle all night long.

Synthetic drugs they can disturb your vital synergies

But hawthorn is a gentle herb to prevent the heart disease

Celebrex may have killed some men But not me, what me worry

With my arthritis kickin' in; just up my dose of curry

Turmeric's antiarthritic As it seems to displace;
     Cyclooxygenase

And if you're overliving, There's one herb you should choose

Milk thistle saves the liver; From the mushrooms and the
     booze.

Compression stockings, atrocities, gimme horse chestnut
     pills

To slow down varicosities; Better than drugs will

We often talk in alphabets, EPO and GLA

Will help to put to rest BPH and PMS

Been taking evening primrose; Two decades more or less
And almost everybody knows, I ain't got PMS

Final Exam (with Answers)

Whattaya take for gout? Celery seed!

For flu? Echinacea!

For high cholesterol? Garlic!

For the liver? Milk thistle!

For the memory? Ginkgo

For arthritis? Turmeric!

For chronic venous insufficiency (CVI)? Horse chestnut!

For the heart? Hawthorn!

For benign prostatic hypertrophy (BPH)? Saw palmetto!

For premenstrual syndrome (PMS)? Evening primrose!

For stress? Kava!

For depression? St. John's wort!

For failing eyesight? Bilberry![35]

Precautions with Herbs

These are terrific herbs, mostly proven very safe. But **never take any herb without first consulting** *with your doctor to see if there are any harmful interactions, either with your condition or with drugs you are taking.*

Kava should not be taken in large amounts or with alcohol or Tylenol because it can hurt the liver. Make sure the brand you buy is made from the root only. Don't take it if you drive; it might make you sleepy and inattentive.

Saint John's wort can give you photosensitivity—an exaggerated response to sun. It should not be mixed with other antidepressants and mood medications, and it can decrease the effectiveness of some pharmaceuticals, including Coumadin and contraceptives. Ask your pharmacist.

Echinacea should not be taken if you have an autoimmune disease or multiple sclerosis, as the jury is still out about it.

Garlic in high doses and **ginkgo** can increase bleeding in people on Coumadin. Garlic could also lower your blood sugar if you are a diabetic—a beneficial side effect, just be aware of it.

As Jim Duke has said, he does not take every herb every day. Instead, keep them at hand when you need them. I like to take my herbs as tinctures: I drop them into hot water and drink them like a tea. Many people prefer capsules. Teabags or loose herbs are fine, but usually not as concentrated and effective. Just make sure you follow the dosage information on the package. In the United States, there is no general standardization of herbs. You have to buy from a reliable source.

Always buy the whole herb, not a patented medicine that takes single ingredients from a plant. The plant has lived with humans for eons; use the wisdom of the whole plant and not a pharmaceutical herb concoction. The only reason manufacturers make these concoctions is because whole plants cannot be patented and not enough profit can be made from them.

And Don't Forget . . .

I want to sneak in a few more herbs that I think are terrific for staying young longer. Here are the herbs I want to add to the list—unfortunately without Jim Duke's poetry.

Stinging Nettle

In Europe, we think that nettle is the single most useful herb. It is often considered a nuisance weed, but it is filled with remarkable substances. Nettle leaves are anti-inflammatory, they are a perfect booster for your immune system, and they also keep hay fever and asthma at bay. (Quit dairy first—you might never even have to take nettle.)

Nettle **root** is good for the prostate: for prostatitis and BPH (benign prostatic hypertrophy), which is a bit of a misnomer because what is *benign* in having to get up twenty times per night for a few drops of urine each time and then needing surgery?

Aloe

I always have aloe plants in the house. They grow well in a pot on the windowsill. The huge, leathery aloe leaves are now also available in health-food stores and supermarkets—looking more as if they could be used for slaying someone than for healing purposes. The little plants you grow yourself are as good as the huge ones you buy. Use the jellylike substance in the middle of the fleshy leaf: Just cut it open and scrape out the gel. The outside tough skin is a powerful and dangerous laxative, in the same forbidden category as senna and *Cascara sagrada*. It is habit-forming and should not be taken other than for a few days and under the supervision of a physician.

I use aloe for two conditions: healing skin wounds (applied to the skin) and soothing the digestive tract—from gums to esophagus to stomach. I swish the undiluted jelly around in my mouth before swallowing it. That way, my gums and my heartburn are treated at the same time. Aloe, besides its healing compounds, contains bitter substances and therefore is a boon for digestion.

Make sure that you don't use aloe on deep wounds. Its healing power is so great that it can close a wound superficially before the deeper-lying tissues have healed, which might get you into trouble because a wound should close from the inside out to prevent pockets of infection.

Ginger

Ginger is a heart-warming medication—that's how I look at it. Whenever you have a cold or feel one coming, ginger in hot water does wonders. It works as a powder as well as freshly cut. My favorite cough tea is made from peppermint, ginger, clove, honeysuckle and horehound.

Ginger is also a wonderful drug against nausea and motion sickness. And it is safe in pregnancy. Ginger might increase bleeding—so be careful if you take Coumadin. Like garlic, it improves diabetes and can therefore lead to too-low blood sugar if you are on diabetes medication. For some people, it increases stomach acidity, which usually is not a problem in the elderly, who often suffer from the opposite—too low stomach acidity.

Living the Good Life: A Portrait of Henrietta

At 84, Henrietta is sharp as a tack and still interested in the world around her. She goes out every day with her walker. At home, she uses a wheelchair most of the time. She wears bright colors and loves to paint, but lately her eyesight is failing, and she considered giving up painting altogether. Instead, she chose to use stronger colors and bigger brushes. She calls it "my blind series." Her flowers look full of life and sunshine.

Henrietta takes part in her art group's exhibitions; she also is the club's treasurer. And she never would give up lunches and chats with her many friends. She lost her husband many years ago, but is close to all four of her children. People like

Henrietta because Henrietta likes people. Once, after a short hospital stay, she told me how wonderful everyone in the hospital had treated her. "The best thing was that I had a *male* nurse, and he washed me up from head to toe—and I just *loved* it." Her laugh is irresistible.

Many times the question of a nursing home has come up. Henrietta showed me her well-organized kitchen and household. It was clear that she did not want to leave the neat home where she has spent most of her life. Her children would have liked her in the safer environment of an assisted-living facility, but Henrietta declined. As her doctor, I discussed the options with her. I was worried about her in a medical emergency. But Henrietta had decided what she wanted: to face things when they came up and enjoy life at home until then. I finally sided with her to stay in her home as long as possible— even if that meant she might fall one day, and help might come too late. "I am ready to leave this life," she said. "I've had a hell of a good life. I just prefer to stay at home."

Henrietta survived several minor medical crises. Then a place opened up at the one assisted-living facility in her town that she liked. She made up her mind and moved within a few days. She proudly showed me around her new place. "They even allow me to host the board meeting for my art club here," she crowed delightedly. Needless to say, she loves the people at the new place, and the people love her.

14

AILMENTS YOU MIGHT FACE AND WHAT TO DO ABOUT THEM

Lifestyle plays a much bigger role in the health of older folks than medical intervention—although I definitely want a surgeon if I break my hip or develop a cancerous growth. Not everybody makes it through the prime of life in good health, however. People have ailments and experience the aches and pains that come "naturally" with the years. I believe you can reduce aches and pains by good eating and exercise. But even if you have a chronic disease—or even a few of them—don't let them stop you. You still can have fun.

Improving Your Odds

Make sure that you take advantage of all the services your doctor has to offer you. Get a yearly physical—it does not guarantee health, but it is one safeguard. And get the following necessary shots:

- **Tetanus.** Everyone should have a tetanus shot every ten years. Remember the date because your doctor might forget it. Tetanus (lockjaw) is a horrible disease, and most of the time it is fatal once it has started. It nearly always leads to a death of pain and agony—and is easily preventable.
- **Pneumococcal vaccination.** Once or twice in your lifetime probably conveys lasting protection. It does not protect you from all pneumonias, but it is still worthwhile.
- **Flu shot (influenza vaccine).** For people over sixty-five or with a disease such as asthma, chronic bronchitis, heart disease or diabetes, a flu shot is a good idea. Unfortunately, the vaccine has to be given every fall, and there is some concern about the repeated mercury dose.

Alphabetical List of Common Ailments

Here are some ailments, listed alphabetically, that might accompany you on your journey through a long life, and a few tips how to avoid or improve them before you reach for the big guns. *Do not take any supplements without first consulting with your doctor for potential side effects or drug interactions.*

Some of the recommendations might seem repetitive, but healthy living is based on a few simple truths—and they cannot be repeated often enough.

Aches and Pains
(See also Arthritis, Chronic Pain, Pain)

Some people claim that when you are over fifty and one morning you wake up and feel no pain, you are dead. I disagree with that statement.

Aches and pains have causes. I don't want to dispute that there can be severe pain from disease, but those "minor" aches and pains that so many people take for granted can be minimized or even eliminated.

Most aches and pains come from three causes:

1. Not enough exercise

2. Too much or the wrong kind of exercise
3. Wrong foods that cause inflammation in the body

Basically, these three points boil down to: Listen to your body. If jogging hurts you, why would you continue doing it?

The biggie, of course, is number one: too little exercise. The right exercise—a healthy mixture between strengthening, balancing and opening—will free your body from most pain. Our joints are meant to be moved and released. Instead, we think age means being hunched down and bent over. Go back to chapter 10 and learn about yoga, tai chi, walking and playing.

Alzheimer's Disease (See also Memory Loss)

Losing mental capacity is very high on the list of what people fear about aging. My mother used to say: "Just push me off the cliff when I lose my marbles," which is really not an option, of course.

Here is what research says about preventing Alzheimer's disease—it comes down to "what's good for your heart, is good for your head":

- **Eat healthfully.** The more green stuff, the more berries, the more different vegetables and fruit and nuts (and perhaps grains) you squeeze into your day, the better.
- **Exercise.** Do things! Move around! Nothing ages you more than sitting at home in front of the TV or computer.
- **Get light into your face and on your body.** Avoid the bad sun rays but gobble up, drink in, relish light. Strip down to naked once a day. Go out in the light for a walk or a hike. It replenishes vitamin D and tells your brain that you still want to be alive. It furnishes you with stimulating things to see, to hear, to smell.
- **Avoid aluminum and coated cookware.**
- **Avoid toxins.** Steer clear of mercury, solvents, pesticides and so on. If you suspect that you might be loaded with pollutants, go on a mild cleanse with stinging nettle, milk thistle and dandelion. But stay away from high colonics and abrasive laxatives to clean out your intestines. If you start eating more healthfully, your body will self-cleanse itself.
- **Use fresh herbs.** Make herb tea and use herbs freely in the kitchen: lemon balm, rosemary, sage, hyssop, cilantro, parsley, mint,

watercress. And use dried herbs, too.

- **Add lime to your diet.** Lime has anti-Alzheimer's potential—herbs and lime contain cholinesterase inhibitor, a powerful compound that is a prime "suspect" in helping your brain synapses to continue functioning.

Arthritis
(See also Aches and Pains, Chronic Pain, Pain)

Arthritis pain is caused by inflammation in the joints, so anything you can do to reduce the inflammation will help. Here are some recommended methods from integrative medicine:

- **Movement.**
  — Physical therapy for mobility and strengthening
  — Gentle yoga
  — The Traditional Chinese exercises tai chi and/or qigong
- **Meditation for relaxation.** See "A Closer Look at Meditation" in chapter 4.
- **Energy and movement therapies.**
  — Acupuncture—recent research supports the use of acupuncture for osteoarthritis of

the knee, and other studies are ongoing.[36]

— Massage, including muscular therapy, shiatsu, trigger point, craniosacral therapy.

— Alexander Technique and Trager® Movement Education.

• **Supplements**[37] **and more.** Consult with your doctor for correct dosage and type.

— **Glucosamine sulfate** was found to be as effective as ibuprofen with fewer adverse reactions. You have to try it for about half a year before you can say it doesn't work in you. Sometimes glucosamine is combined with chondroitin sulfate. The evidence for chondroitin is not that strong so far—and usually glucosamine alone is cheaper.

— **Capsaicin,** a compound prepared from hot peppers, reduces pain in arthritis patients if used as a gel or ointment. It is a bit messy, but it works just fine. Don't get it in your eyes—it burns!

— **Pulsed electromagnetic field stimulation** by a device called a TENS unit, a method of physical medicine. A TENS unit machine costs about $100, and works well in muscle spasm-induced pain.

• **Healing foods.** Always remember the food

connection: food allergies and intolerances can lead to chronic inflammation in your body. My best recommendation is to rotate the foods that you eat, and eat a diet as varied as possible, high in vegetables and herbs. (See chapter 8, Nourish Your Body.) Following are healing foods for arthritis:

— Pineapple.
— Broccoli.
— Lots of fresh vegetables. Jim Duke's "arthritis soup" includes cabbage, string beans, celery, stinging nettle leaves, carrots, asparagus, dandelion root, spinach, eggplant, chicory, garlic, turmeric, licorice, evening primrose seeds, ground red pepper, white mustard, flaxseed, sarsaparilla, fenugreek and lemon juice.[38]
— Seawater fish.

• **Herbs.** Botanist James A. Duke, author of *The Green Pharmacy*, recommends the following herbs for arthritis:[39]

— Garlic
— Ginger
— Oregano
— Rosemary

— Stinging nettle
— Turmeric
— Willow bark

Cellulite

Cellulite is a disease of wrong foods combined with too little movement. So, shun dairy, sugar and white starches and shake it, baby! Daily dry brushing of the thighs with a loofah sponge or a soft brush will help, too.

Chronic Bronchitis, COPD, Respiratory Disease

Try the following approaches for relief from chronic bronchitis, COPD, and other respiratory diseases. (For relentless, violent, bloody or pussy cough, see your doctor immediately.)

- **Stop all dairy.** Dairy is a mucus-producing food.
- **Quit smoking.**
- **Drink plenty of water.**
- **Reduce phlegm.** Try these herbs:
  — Anise seeds
  — Cloves

- — Fennel seeds
- — Licorice root (not licorice candy!)
- — Linden flowers
- — Meadowsweet flowers
- — Mullein flowers
- — Plantain leaves, herb
- — Thyme leaves
- **Soothe cough.** The following can help eliminate cough:
  - — Coltsfoot leaves
  - — Cordyceps mushroom
  - — Eucalyptus
  - — Fennel
  - — Fenugreek
  - — Iceland moss
  - — Marshmallow root
  - — Thyme
- **Rinse nose with saltwater.** Cough can be triggered by sinusitis. Learn to rinse your nose with saltwater. (See "Colds and Flu" for instructions on how to do this.)
- **Steam inhalations.** Use chamomile, essential oil of pine or Vick's.
- **Breathing exercises.** These can be very beneficial. Discuss this with your physician.
- **Yoga.** Practicing yoga opens the lungs.

- **Daily outside walks.** Walk for exercise, light exposure and fresh air.
- **Healthful nutrition.** Eat a diet high in vegetables and fruit.

Chronic Pain
(See also Aches and Pains, Arthritis, Pain)

If a pain has settled so deeply into your body that you want to ask your physician for stronger painkillers or surgery, it might be worthwhile to explore some bodywork methods first. Unfortunately, you might have to pay for them out of your pocket—but this is money well spent. (American Western Life Insurance Company is one of the few that covers many alternative health services.) Bodywork does not build up strength and stamina, but it helps you relax, let go and open. It addresses musculoskeletal pain from a holistic—whole body—perspective. Here are some types of bodywork to consider:

- Trager approach
- Chiropractic
- Shiatsu

- Chinese massage
- Feldenkrais
- Swedish massage
- Alexander Technique
- Rolfing
- Deep-tissue massage
- Thai massage

In all these methods, word-of-mouth referral is the most valuable, so ask around. ***And check with your doctor before embarking on any of these!***

Colds and Flu

A cold is a nuisance, but the flu can be deadly. Asthma, autoimmune diseases, cancer, chronic bronchitis (smoking!), diabetes and obesity make you more prone to all kinds of infections.

Here are ways to prevent colds and the flu:

- Get your flu shot, but know that the vaccine is not foolproof.
- Wash your hands frequently.
- Rinse your nose with saltwater once or twice daily during the season (see page 135 for instructions).
- Eat lots of vegetables.

- Have chicken soup ready, preferably homemade.
- Take a daily walk in all weather, and take a cold shower after each warm one.
- Avoid undue stress; get enough sleep.
- Nibble on a clove of garlic.
- In a bad pandemic, wear a face mask and stay away from people.

And once it has hit you:

- Keep low for a few days and sleep early and long to give your immune system a chance to heal your body.
- Drink tons of hot fluid—a lemon or lime, squeezed into a glass of hot water, is one of the best remedies. Forgo the sugar or honey.
- Try hot blueberry soup. Barely cover the contents of one package of frozen blueberries with water; bring to a fast boil, then allow to cool enough to eat the whole concoction of berries and liquid. This gives you vitamins and minerals to help fight infection. And the blue color in the blueberries kills infectious agents, too. (This soup is also good for acute stomach flu and urinary tract infections.) Hot elderberry soup is good, too—but hard to come by. You can buy the elderberry juice as Sambucol®,

but blueberries are much cheaper.

- Eat only if you are hungry; nobody starves in a week. The less you eat, the better your body can concentrate on defending itself.

- Herbal teas that might help a cold: ginger, peppermint, linden, elderberry flowers.

- Keep on nibbling the garlic and rinsing your nose with saltwater—many times per day if needed.

- My recipe for a cough tea: peppermint, ginger (fresh or dried), cloves, honeysuckle and horehound. (Keep these ingredients on hand because once you get sick it is too late to chase them down.)

- Unsweetened elderberry concentrate and black cherry juice have been proven to work in colds.

- And please, don't smoke—you are setting your lungs up for an invasion of the viral and bacterial hordes!

- The four herbs that I take (as extracts in hot water) when flu hits me (take as directed on the bottle—about one dropper full three times a day) are: echinacea, osha, olive leaf extract and pau d'arco.

Know when you are too sick to go it alone at

home. If you suspect you might have pneumonia (prolonged or high fevers, shortness of breath and/or pains on deep breathing), check yourself into an emergency room.

SINUS IRRIGATION FOR EAR, THROAT AND UPPER RESPIRATORY INFECTIONS

Sinus irrigation, also known as sinus wash or lavage, is a simple procedure that can increase drainage of the sinuses. For seasonal allergies, sinus irrigation can remove pollen from the nose. It can also help with upper respiratory infections and colds and be useful for certain types of asthma that include upper respiratory symptoms. It has been recommended by physicians for decades, and its use dates further back in traditional Eastern practices.

The technique uses an "isotonic saline solution," which has a similar salt concentration to body fluids. To make the solution, you will need the following:

1 teaspoon salt—kosher, canning, pickling, or sea salt is preferable to table salt

16 ounces water (0.47 liter or 1 U.S. pint), at room temperature

Instructions:

1. Mix the ingredients together.
2. Insert solution into a clean rubber-topped dropper. If unavailable, an ear syringe, neti pot (a tea pot for the nose), or clean hand can be used. You can also wash a

dropper from an empty tincture bottle.

3. Pour some of the solution into the palm of your hand. Sniff it up. Continue until the glass is empty. It feels like drowning in the ocean—but it only runs down in your mouth. Then spit it out.

Precautions and Risks: Do not swallow the salty liquid; it can increase blood pressure.

Constipation

Constipation is a civilization disease—and can be counteracted with:

- Lots of fresh fruits and vegetables.
- Regular exercises, especially walking, and all practices that focus on your abs.
- Plenty of filtered water, warm or hot.
- Try fenugreek, flaxseed, psyllium, raisins, prunes, prune juice or figs. Avoid harsh laxatives such as senna, *Cascara sagrada*, aloe.
- One cup of coffee in the morning might work as a gentle laxative. More is not better!

Don't forget to follow the urge. Go when your body wants to go. If you delay, your body will retrieve water from your colon. As a result, the feces will become harder, more difficult to expel.

Depression

For many people, aging goes hand in hand with depression. They have no outlook, no interests, no curiosity, no attachments. One doctor I know said that to be healthy and happy a person needs three things: something to do, something to look forward to, and someone to love.

Get professional help for depression, but also know that antidepressant medication can give you a host of new ailments. Your best option is to combine initial pharmaceutical therapy with psychotherapy and the ideas from this book to build up a healthy, meaningful life. The following suggestions can be especially helpful:

- Exercise produces endorphins, natural "feel-good" hormones, and research has shown exercise to be as effective as medication in treating mild to moderate depression.
- Saint John's wort is active against mild to moderate depression, but you have to know its side-effects (like photosensitivity) and interactions with medications (ask your doctor or pharmacist).
- Go out daily, preferably before noon, to fight the winter blues (and the blues, period) with

light exposure and movement. Both increase
endorphins in your blood.

- Get involved with people who are worse off
  than you. Look for opportunities to volunteer: Read for sick youngsters or blind people,
  help build houses for the poor. Use whatever
  skills you bring to give freely to the people
  who need it. One of our friends, after his
  spouse died and he had gone through grieving
  for a few years, joined an international rescue
  commission and now offers his help at an
  interesting project in Armenia. His life is not
  yet over because he has found a new purpose.

- Try licorice (the real stuff, not the candy). It
  is an immune booster but also contains many
  antidepressive compounds.

- Take fish oil capsules regularly, or evening
  primrose and/or walnuts, pumpkin and sun-
  flower seeds. I suspect that all raw nuts are good
  for your brain—just beware of food allergies.

- Other herbs to add to your food: thyme,
  purslane, ginger (preferably unsugared),
  ginkgo, ginseng (not if you have high blood
  pressure), lamb's quarters, rosemary and pig-
  weed. (I thank Jim Duke for these suggestions
  from his *Green Pharmacy*.)

• Eating a diet high in carbohydrates makes some people feel better, probably because of their high vitamin B content and their effect on tryptophan levels. The drawback is that if you pack on pounds from this diet, you might feel worse about yourself. Restrict your whole grains and legumes to breakfast.

Diabetes

A diet based on vegetables, as proposed in this book, and regular exercise will prevent type 2 diabetes. Many of my patients have had spectacular success with this approach.

Ask your doctor to check your A1c (glycohemoglobin) with each visit, as it is a powerful motivator to continue your efforts. If it is 6.0 or higher, you have diabetes. "Natural" physicians consider values above 5.0 as pre-diabetes, a condition not optimal in spite of conventional medicine declaring it *normal.*

You know that diabetes is a disease of too much sugar, right? But did you also know that bad fats, proteins (meats and poultry) and even smoking can trigger diabetes? They produce glycotoxins. Glycotoxins have been implicated as one of the key causes of diabetes and—together with free radicals—of aging. With a diet mostly based on vegetables, you avoid many glycotoxins.

Here is a list of the five foods most laced with glycotoxins that should be avoided:

- Broiled hot dogs
- Oven-fried chicken
- Oven-fried fish
- McDonald's Chicken McNuggets
- Broiled chicken breast

And you thought that chicken was healthful, or that broiling was superior! We all have to relearn, it seems. In a good soup—like grandma's!—the temperature never goes much higher than boiling water, and it is one of the healthiest meals you can have.

Dizziness, Frequent Falls, Loss of Balance, Vertigo

Major fractures due to falls are frequently fatal in the elderly. Studies have shown that the regular practice of tai chi, a series of slow, flowing exercise movements originating from Traditional Chinese Medicine, improves balance, coordination and strength in the elderly and helps to prevent falls.[40, 41]

Yoga, another mind-body practice, also improves

balance, posture and flexibility. Know that many diseases can cause loss of balance. See your doctor.

Eye Problems

More Americans are facing blindness than ever before—due to the aging population, and also due to unhealthful lifestyles. These are the four most common causes—in the order of their frequency:

1. Cataracts: more than 20 million
2. Diabetic retinopathy: more than 5 million
3. Glaucoma: more than 2 million
4. Age-related macular degeneration: 1.6 million

The causes are different, but here is what you can do:

- See an eye doctor (ophthalmologist) regularly.
- Eat a healthful diet with vegetables, fruit and berries, seafood and nuts.
- For macular degeneration, you might benefit from a bilberry/zinc preparation.
- Do not use high-dose vitamins without discussing it with a knowledgeable physician.
- Exercise moderately but regularly to oxygenate your body.

Fatigue, Daytime Sleepiness, Chronic Weakness

Eat better, exercise and follow the rules against insomnia (see "Insomnia"). If you sleep well at night, you will experience less daytime fatigue. Also:

- Have your doctor check your thyroid and your vitamin B_{12} level.
- Scrutinize your schedule if you are overdoing things. Sometimes, even fun things turn out to create stress.
- Unfortunately, fatigue is a symptom of many diseases. If lifestyle changes do not improve the situation soon, check with your doctor to find out what is wrong. A healthy organism is not constantly tired.

Gout

Most gout sufferers are men, so not all is the fault of a bad diet. But good nutrition still is the key to a goutfree life. A healthful diet also helps to avoid the dreaded kidney stones that may accompany gout. Other things that can help:

- **Use an ice pack** in an acute attack for not longer than fifteen minutes over the affected joint.

- **Adequate water intake.** This is most important: seven cups per day (warm)—more with exercise.

- **Nutrition.** Eat a healthy, fresh, balanced, seasonal, preferably local, moderate, organic diet. Legumes (peas, beans, lentils, garbanzos) are high-protein foods. Reduce your portions of meat, poultry and fish. Avoid:

  — Alcoholic beverages, especially beer
  — Anchovies
  — Asparagus
  — Cacao
  — Cauliflower
  — Chocolate
  — Coffee
  — Cola
  — Dairy
  — Deli meats
  — Fish roes
  — Herring
  — Lobster
  — Meat extracts (broth, consommé, gravies)
  — Mushrooms
  — Mussels

— Organ meats (liver, kidneys, sweetbreads)

— Sardines

— Shrimp

— Spinach

— Spirulina

— Tea

Good for you:

— Berries

— Fish oil

— Flaxseed

— Fruit

— Nuts

— Olive oil

— Salmon (but not in huge amounts because of possible mercury overload)

— Tempeh

— Tofu

— Vegetables (most)

— Whole grains

• **Exercise.** Exercise is very important. Uric acid is stored in gout—and the more movement, the sluggish your metabolism. Start after an acute gout attack and be easy on your joints—for instance, try "gentle running" instead of jogging. If you have an exercise machine—any, it doesn't matter which kind—use it every day for two minutes. No excuses! If you have none, walk stairs briskly for two minutes.

- **Reduce your weight.** But do this slowly (if it applies) because sudden weight loss (or gain) can elicit a gout attack.

- **Take a daily cold shower.** Take a cold shower after the warm one to increase circulation.

- **Herbs.** Try this tea: horsetail, rose hips, juniper berries, birch leaves and nettle leaves in about equal amounts and mixed. Bring one teaspoon to a short boiling. Let steep for another ten minutes. Drink this once a day for three weeks, then take a break for at least three weeks.

- **Balancing your life.** A healthy balance between rest and movement is probably the most important point for gout. Get enough sleep before midnight. Don't let your body get into a run-down state.

Hair Loss

Find out if it is just male- (or female-) pattern baldness or a disease.

- Have your doctor check your hormones.

- Stop all harsh hair treatments like curling/ uncurling and chemical dyes. Henna is a safer product and comes in shades from blonde to black.
- Start healthful eating now with lots of vege- tables and a reasonable amount of protein.
- Sugar seems to have a detrimental effect on hair—as does alcohol (which is a sugar). I can often spy alcoholics by their lusterless hair.
- Exercise aerobically because it will bring oxygen to your hair roots.
- Once a month, especially in the winter, treat your hair and scalp (and your whole body) to an oil bath with sesame or olive oil. Be extra careful not to burn yourself. You need about a cup of warm (not hot!) oil. In the shower, smear it all over your body, without the water running. Wait about ten minutes, then sham- poo your hair two to three times. This oil treatment nourishes your scalp and gives your hair shine and heaviness on a dry winter day.
- Use a good olive oil in your cooking and on salads.
- Eat nuts, which contain minerals and vita- mins for healthy hair.
- Saw palmetto berries and stinging nettle cap- sules both give you full hair (but not as much as a hair transplant).

- The healthful diet described in this book will help your hair as well.
- On and off, drink a tea made with the herb horsetail. Not too often, however; it is harsh on the kidneys.

Heartburn, GERD, Reflux, Dyspepsia, Stomach Pain, Gastritis

The causes for stomach ailments are myriad. A conventional physician should make a diagnosis. He or she should look for (among other things):

- Food allergies
- Gluten intolerance
- *Helicobacter pylori*
- High gastrin levels
- Low acidity/high acidity
- Parasites

But if your doctor can come up with nothing better than pharmaceutical pills (which sometimes are a godsend!), you can still try these tips.

Avoid these:
- Antacids (they make the problem worse in the long run)
- Aspirin

- Big meals (try several small meals a day)
- Carbonated beverages
- Chocolate
- Coffee
- Dairy
- Eating in a lying position (in bed, on the couch)
- Excess meats, poultry and game
- Fatty foods
- Fluids with meals (drink half an hour before and one and a half hours afterward)
- Late-night meals (do not eat after dinner; have dinner early)
- Nightshades
- Peppermint
- Salty food, especially if diagnosed with *H. pylori*
- Smoking
- Strong spices
- Sugars and starches
- Tea (black and green)

Different measures help different people. Try these:

- DGL (licorice) before meals
- Digestive enzymes

- Probiotics (acidophilus preparations)
- Head of bed should be slightly elevated
- Mastic gum extract
- Plantain banana, banana, slippery elm, marshmallow, calendula can be soothing to the GI tract
- Zinc-containing foods: seafood, legumes, whole grains
- Vitamin A-containing foods: liver, eggs, butter, cream and cod liver oil; and beta carotenes (precursors of vitamin A): dark green and orange-yellow vegetables
- Bitter herbs such as dandelion, gentiana, artichoke, milk thistle, arugula, chicory, dill, parsley—preferably before or at the beginning of the meal (they jumpstart the digestive juices)
- Bioflavonoids: they give the colors to fruit and vegetables
- High fiber
- Herbs against *H. pylori*: aloe vera, astragalus, cabbage juice (about $1/2$–1 liter throughout the day), chamomile, clove, DGL licorice, garlic, goldenseal, marshmallow, neem, pau d'arco, thyme, slippery elm

Heart Disease

A heart-healthy diet and life is what this book is all about—the same with the moderate exercise I recommend here. In addition to diet and exercise, try to:

- Reduce stress by learning yoga, tai chi and/or meditation.
- Think about what is important in your life. Think more about *doing* and *being* than about *having*.
- Practice forgiveness.
- Open your heart to people worse off than you.

Hemorrhoids

A diet high in fiber—see my vegetable-based suggestions in chapter 8—prevents hemorrhoids. Also, plants provide vessel-wall-strengthening compounds like rutin and flavonoids. In addition to a plant-based diet, you should:

- Use good oils (like olive oil) in your food.
- Never stand or sit too long. If you have to stand, shift from one leg to the other constantly (to activate the venous pump in your legs). Put up your feet as often as possible to let the blood return.

- End all your hot showers with a few seconds of cold water. Let the water run between your crease. This has a soothing action on your hemorrhoids.
- Do a cold sitz bath with a few inches of cold water in the tub. Sit for a few minutes. Terminate when it gets uncomfortable. (This practice is contraindicated in urinary tract infection and fever situations—confer with your doctor.)
- Follow the recommendations in "Constipation," as excessive straining promotes hemorrhoids.

High Blood Pressure

Along with diabetes, high blood pressure is a typical civilization disease—and 95 percent avoidable. Try the following recommendations:

- Drink plenty of water.
- Learn to de-stress through daily walking, meditation, exercise, yoga and/or tai chi.
- Avoid processed foods.
- Eat foods good for you: olive oil (in moderation), onions and garlic, and a high-potassium diet of fruit and vegetables (spruced up with fish three times a week, and meat once a week).

- Avoid salt.
- Learn to manage anger.
- Have a few quiet minutes every day to yourself. (The act of speaking elevates your blood pressure).
- Don't suppress your feelings: voice them and get rid of them.
- Slowly but surely (not quickly!) approach your ideal weight with healthy lifestyle choices.
- If your job/boss/co-workers are causing your high blood pressure, start thinking about a change of occupation. What would you rather do? What are your skills, your forte? Frustration on the job can lead to heart attacks—that is why heart attacks peak on Mondays.
- Most workouts are good for high blood pressure, except heavy weightlifting and other isometric exercises.
- Stop all alcohol except for one small glass of wine or beer per day. If you have difficulties giving it up, get professional help.
- Quit smoking—you should have quit long ago, and every day makes it worse.
- Consider buying a blood pressure machine and check your blood pressure regularly.

High Cholesterol

Very few people have a truly *inborn* lipid imbalance—most of us have the diet-related kind. So read chapter 8 on nutrition, implement the changes to your diet and start exercise. No pill can buy you health—only your own effort will. Aim for your ideal weight and Body Mass Index. As author Laura Lewis says, "You can't change your matter if you don't change your mind."[42]

Hot Flashes and Other Menopausal Symptoms

Discuss this with your doctor first, but most women do fine with these four herbs (take a dropper of each in a big cup of hot water once to twice a day):

- Black cohosh
- Ginkgo (unless you are taking an anticoagulant such as Coumadin)
- Red clover
- Wild yam

And eat healthfully, exercise in moderation and make your relationships work. If all this does not improve your symptoms, ask your physician to add a tiny bit of natural (bio-identical) hormones.

Impotence, Loss of Desire and Missing Orgasms (in Women)

I cannot stress the importance of a common-sense approach to this widespread (and widely feared) ailment.

- Confer with your doctor because more serious disease has to be ruled out before you can embark on self-healing. Make sure to have your hormones tested.
- Eat healthfully.
- Do some daily exercise.
- Keep clean. Nothing turns on lovers more than a freshly bathed and groomed partner.
- For women: ginkgo, ginger, ginseng (not with high blood pressure or anticoagulants), wild yam, damiana.
- For men: saw palmetto, ginkgo, ginger, ginseng (last three not with high blood pressure or anticoagulants), yohimbe (as an extract—called yohimbine hydrochloride—rather than the whole plant because the whole plant has side effects on the heart and the nervous system).
- For both: aromatherapy. A few drops of an essential oil sprinkled on a lamp ring can turn

a Spartan bedroom into a lascivious boudoir. Never ever swallow essential oils—internally they are toxic, even in small amounts.

- Essential oils are even too concentrated to put directly on your skin, but try a few drops in olive oil, and massage your partner with it. Start at the feet. . . .
- Explore tantric yoga.

Incontinence, Urinary (Women)

Let your doctor decide if you have stress or urge incontinence—some people have a mixture. But before you follow his or her recommendations for surgery (which should be the last resort), try these things first:

- Have your doctor check you for chronic bladder infection.
- Stop all bladder irritants (especially for urge incontinence):
  — Cigarettes and coffee
  — Medical drugs (ask your pharmacist or look up each pill on the Internet)
  — Foods to which you might be allergic
- For stress incontinence, walk daily, preferably on hilly and uneven terrain. It exercises your

pelvic muscles. Do Kegel exercises: When you urinate, try to stop the flow. The muscles that stop the flow are your pelvic floor muscles. Once you have pinpointed those muscles, you can contract them wherever you are—standing at the bus stop, waiting in line, sitting at your desk. Start with three muscle contractions; work up to three, five times a day. It is tedious—but beats surgery. Biofeedback can help you locate those muscles if you have a hard time.

- Electrical stimulation therapy (with a vaginal or anal probe) has improved incontinence and has been recommended by the National Institute of Health, as outlandish as the idea might seem.

- Reduce abdominal fat. That is the number two factor making your pelvic floor muscles sag (number one, is of course, childbearing—and we wouldn't want to miss that one!).

- Wear comfortable clothes that don't hamper your belly's freedom.

Insomnia

Practice good sleep hygiene:

- Go to bed around 10 P.M.

- Read something relaxing.
- Go to sleep before 11 P.M. (between 11 P.M. and 1 A.M. every night, the body makes major repairs—if you're sleeping, that is).
- Don't drink alcohol to help you sleep—it actually makes you wake up in the middle of the night, when the alcohol wears off.
- Don't sleep more than nine hours per day (naptime included).
- Have your bedroom as dark as possible because light signals your inner eye that it is time to get up. (Getting up with the sun actually might be a good idea—a big reason for insomnia is that we have lost our natural rhythms since the invention of electric light.)
- Protect yourself from noise as much as possible. White noise or a CD of a waterfall or rain sounds can drown out intruding noises.
- Don't fret when you can't sleep. Read a book or keep a diary or a dream journal.
- Avoid TV shortly before sleep and remove the TV from your bedroom.
- Make sure your bed and covers are comfortable. A firm mattress is usually the best.
- Don't work in your bed or bedroom, as that makes it harder to let go of what is on your mind.

- Fall asleep and awaken to soothing music.
- Work out during the day so that you get physically tired.
- If a full bladder wakes you up, avoid drinking within two hours of bedtime—and take saw palmetto berries to shrink your prostate gland if you are a man.
- Avoid caffeine after noon—or completely, if you are sensitive to its effects (some over-the-counter pain medications also contain caffeine).
- Ask your doctor and your pharmacist whether any of your prescription medications might be adding to your sleep problem.
- Have an early dinner—many people sleep better if they have their last meal before six o'clock. Make sure it contains some protein to last, but the bulk should consist of soothing carbohydrates.
- Do not eat at night (unless you are a diabetic on a regimen). Interestingly, a solid breakfast can prevent you from raiding your fridge at night.
- Sleep with your window open if you live in a quiet area.
- Keep the temperature in your bedroom below 60 degrees F.

- Try aromatherapy. Put a drop of essential oil (lavender, chamomile, jasmine, neroli [bitter orange], rose or marjoram) on a bulb ring. You will fall asleep while happily inhaling. (Be sure you don't have allergies.)
- Never fall asleep without making up with your partner.

Liver Spots

Try lemon juice—dab it on your skin whenever you use it in the kitchen. But first consult your physician to make sure that they are liver spots— not skin cancer.

Memory Loss (See also Alzheimer's Disease)

Certain serious diseases come with memory loss, so you should see a physician to rule those out. Non-Alzheimer's memory loss is defined as the "normal" cognitive impairment that comes with aging.

Causes of memory loss, other than aging, include (not a complete list):

- Atherosclerosis
- Cancer
- Depression

- Diabetes
- Drinking (Avoid substances that nibble away at your brain such as alcoholic beverages in excess, recreational drugs, medicinal drugs that are not absolutely necessary.)
- Head trauma in the past
- High blood pressure
- Homocysteine, elevated
- Infection
- Parathyroid disease
- Sleep apnea
- Smoking
- Thyroid disease
- Vitamin B12 deficiency

I doubt that normal aging has to be accompanied by memory loss. Here is how to prevent it:

- Train your brain! Learn new skills. (I know somebody who took up playing piano in his late seventies. I myself began cello lessons at the age of fifty-seven.) Do crossword puzzles, read books, take classes, make new friends, go hiking—show your brain that it is still needed.
- Exercise, because that is the way to get oxygen into your body (and your brain).

- Sleep with your window open.
- Vegetables and fruit should be the most important part of your diet.
- Ginkgo biloba is the best-researched herb against dementia (but do not take it if you are on Coumadin).
- Fish oil should be taken for its anti-inflammatory properties (but do not take it if you are on Coumadin).
- Turmeric is one of the spices in curry. Use it frequently, either alone or in a curry mixture.

Osteoporosis

A diet high in vegetables, herbs and fruit will build up strong bones—just as our predecessors, the cavemen and women, had. Cavemen had no dairy cows, but they ate large amounts of plant food and roamed the savannah all day. Take their lifestyle as a model to build strong bones.

Vegetables and whole grains (if you have no problems with grain) also make for a healthy bowel flora—the myriad of good bacteria that help us digest also help us prevent bone loss. Incorporate the following:

- Healthful diet with vegetables, fruit and herbs.
- Regular weight-bearing exercise—such as walking.
- Walk outside daily because the sun promotes production of vitamin D under your skin, which helps calcium absorption. (Consider taking a vitamin D supplement during the winter months.)
- Probiotics (Acidophilus preparation).
- Black and green tea (for their flavonoids contents).

Avoid:
- Dairy
- Soft drinks
- Cigarettes
- Alcohol (more than a glass per day)

If you think you need a calcium supplement (which you won't need if you eat healthfully), choose one that is sugar-free.

Overweight, Obesity

See chapter 9, Painless Weight Loss.

Pain
(See also Aches and Pains, Arthritis, Chronic Pain)

Say you get a headache in the late afternoon. You can pop a pill. Or you can find out what causes the pain and devise a plan. Stress? Go for a short walk. Tired? Take a nap. Too much TV? Do some gentle yoga and release your tight muscles. Had Oreos for lunch? Plan for a healthful dinner with lots of veggies. Too much computer? Get down on your mat for a few minutes of gentle yoga or work out on your rowing machine. Nervous tension? Schedule a massage (or exchange a massage with your partner). Anxiety? Breathe in and out and release your fears.

Pain is there for a reason. But not all pain announces a life-threatening disease. Catch the little pain before it develops into a huge problem. Listen to the pain, attend to it, focus on it. Pain is the language of your body telling you that something is wrong. Before everything else, listen to your body.

One of my patients had very bad plantar fasciitis. We found out that she had some food allergies that had triggered the fasciitis, and she was already working on her nutrition. But she was extremely busy as a professional with a family and didn't have much time to pamper herself. She felt she should try foot massage, but was just too tired. One evening, as she scrambled into bed after another exhausting day, the soles of her feet hurt so excruciatingly that, without having planned this, she heard herself addressing her feet: "I'm really, really sorry. I know I have neglected you, my feet. I promise tomorrow I will do something for you. You deserve better." When she described the episode to me, she lingered on how sheepish she felt. She was such a no-nonsense person. Yet this deep-felt compassion for her poor feet had suddenly broken out of her. "Imagine my surprise next morning when I got up, and all the pain was gone. It was as if my feet just needed to hear my regrets so that the results of the better diet could kick in." To this day, her plantar fasciitis has not returned.

Parkinson's Disease

The reasons for Parkinson's (aside from a genetic disposition) are still unclear. Since the ancient physicians never described it (and they would not have missed such an obvious disease), we have to assume it is a modern disease, somehow linked to our lifestyles. Here are some recommendations I have derived from clinical experience:

- Eat a healthful diet with lots of fresh vegetables. I have seen people who have developed Parkinson's while eating lopsided faddish diets of canned foods only or meals served overcooked and unvaried in institutions.

- If you can manage, choose an uneven surface for walking. A Chinese study recently has shown that it brings major benefit for your muscles, balance and brain function to negotiate cobblestones, pebbles or a similar uneven ground like in the woods.[43]

- Have your blood tested for mercury and lead.

- Go on a detox with milk thistle and stinging nettle.

- Consider a cleansing fast.

- Go outdoors daily and show your face to the light.

- Make use of Trager® Movement Education and other bodywork.

- Walk with the help of a cane or a walker—but walk, walk, walk.

Prostate Ailments

Your prostate likes heart-healthy foods and hates to be sat on. If you impose on your prostate gland the lifestyle of a couch potato or a workaholic, your prostate reacts in three ways: with inflammation (prostatitis), with enlargement BPH (benign prostatic hypertrophy) or with cancer. Some prostate cancer runs in families (especially where there is also breast cancer in women).

My recommendations for a healthy prostate include:

- Eat healthily with plenty of vegetables and herbs, always different ones so that you get your daily load of antioxidants, vitamins and minerals essential for prostate health. All the essentials for prostate health (zinc, boron, selenium, lycopene, beta carotenes, vitamin B_2, vitamin E) are present in a diet consisting of fruit and vegetables, nuts, whole grains and seafood.
- Leave out dairy and be stingy with meat and poultry. Avoid all processed foods.
- Walk daily. Your prostate just loves the gentle massaging it gets from walking because it is located between your legs.
- Walk outdoors because your prostate is grate-

ful for the vitamin D that the light induces in your skin with light exposure.

- Take saw palmetto berries daily for prophylaxis if you are over forty.
- If you are having prostate problems already, add *Pygeum africanum*, stinging nettle root and pumpkin seeds to the saw palmetto.
- Avoid beer and liquor. Wine in moderation seems to be fine, especially red wine that is high in resveratrol. But grapes are loaded with resveratrol, too. Buy organic or wash them very carefully before eating.
- Drink green tea.

Smoking (Quitting)

One out of ten smokers will develop lung cancer but nine out of ten will get emphysema, the horrible disease where you don't get in enough breath to even brush your teeth. Don't let it come to that end stage: Quit now and let the healing begin. Get professional help from your physician. Here are some hints:

- Set a date, tell all your friends and family, and on that day *quit*.
- Remove all cigarettes and ashtrays from your

environment. Throw them away. No hand-me-downs: They are not good for anybody.

- Distance yourself from people who want to hold you back.
- Develop a plan for what to do if you are tempted to smoke: Have chewing gum at hand, go for a walk, call up a friend who accompanies you on your smoking cessation.
- Get the help of a spiritual source. You don't have to go it alone.
- Learn from previous trials. Instead of berating yourself that you failed, ask yourself what you learned and how *not* to do it. Alcohol is one of the frequent reasons people fall back. Avoid drinking/smoking situations: Start a new habit. For instance, if you always lit a cigarette after sex, try to eat an apple or an orange, and share it with your partner.
- Develop a taste for fruit and vegetables because those are the foods that most smokers lack.
- Accompany your smoking cessation by the apple cure: Eat as many apples in the first three days of quitting as you can. The acidity of the apples might aggravate the chronic inflammation in your stomach that stems from smoking—basically, you cannot eat apples and

smoke at the same time. If apples are too tax-ing, eat plenty of cooked vegetables.

- Your physician can help with the patch, nicotine gum or other nicotine preparations. He or she also could prescribe Wellbutrin as an anxiolytic (helping with anxieties), but know you could end up hooked on that medication instead.

- Learn meditation and breathing techniques.

- Lobelia is an herbal remedy used by native Americans. Because it is rather toxic, ask your physician to help you with its use.

- If you fall back to smoking, congratulate yourself for at least having tried. After a few weeks, try again. I don't care if you've tried it twenty or forty times before, one day you will make it.

- Don't allow yourself to smoke in your home—force yourself to go outside.

- Never smoke around children; they suffer most from secondary smoke and also should not see you as a bad role model.

- Find out what keeps you smoking: Boredom? Nervousness? Shyness? Stress? Fear of getting overweight? Constipation? Go on a quest and come to the bottom of your fears—then try quitting again.

- Remember that you will always be in danger, even after quitting. A single puff can get you back into the habit—even after many years.

Stress

For successful aging, you need some healthful stress but not bad stress. So which one is healthful? You decide! You might thrive on something that would throw off other people. (Refer to chapter 4, Letting Go of Bad Stress.) Stress-reducing suggestions include:

- Learn a relaxation technique like meditation, yoga, tai chi.
- Take a relaxing bath with aromatherapy.
- Take a "breather"—breathe deeply, gently for five minutes.
- Go for a walk. My beloved grandfather always took his hat and went for a walk when my volatile grandmother lost her temper. He was the most calming and caring influence in my life.
- Get a massage—or give one.

Stroke

If you have had a stroke already, get all the help you can from:

- Acupuncture
- Exercise—every little bit helps
- Healthful nutrition, including drinking plenty of water
- Physical therapy
- Tai chi
- Trager massage and other forms of bodywork (see Arthritis)
- Yoga

Do not give up because the effects of stroke are often reversible. If stroke runs in your family or if you have been told that you are at risk for it, work on these points for prevention:

- Lower your blood pressure (see High Blood Pressure).
- Drink enough fluid in the form of water or herbal teas.
- Exercise regularly—follow my easy suggestions in chapter 10 on exercise.
- Eat healthfully with plenty of fruit and vegetables. Among others, folate and potassium in

a plant-based diet help lower blood pressure. Go slow on animal meats and fats (chickens are animals, too—fish are more healthful) for a healthy cholesterol level.

- Avoid herbs that might increase your blood pressure:
  — Ginseng
  — Licorice (except DGL)
  — Motherwort
  — Rosemary
- Seaweeds help lower blood pressure, too (if not eaten in huge amounts—they are salty). Use them instead of salt.
- Herbs to take (as a tea, capsules, extract):
  — Chamomile
  — Evening primrose
  — Garlic
  — Ginger
  — Hawthorn
  — Hyssop
  — Lemon balm
  — Parsley
  — Passionflower (also a good "sleeping pill")
  — Skullcap
  — Valerian (also a good "sleeping pill")
  — Yarrow

Thyroid Disease

Hypothyroidism (a sluggish thyroid gland) gets more frequent as we get older. Symptoms are:

- Brittle nails
- Change in menstrual periods
- Constipation
- Fatigue
- Feeling cold constantly
- Hair loss
- Jowls
- Loss of sexual desire
- Memory loss
- Muscle aches
- Muscle weakness
- Puffiness around the eyes
- Weight gain

Once you have been diagnosed with hypothyroidism, you will have to take pills every day. You should also:

- Eat vegetables and fruit daily.
- Find ways to incorporate seaweed into your diet (sprinkle it over salads, soups and stews).
- Avoid dairy.
- Avoid exposure to pollution.

- Take a probiotic (acidophilus preparation).
- Take fish oil capsules (discuss with your physician first).
- Take saw palmetto berries extract.

Ulcers (Skin), Pressure Ulcers

Ulcers have different causes, but it usually comes down to not enough movement and/or faulty nutrition. For pressure ulcers, in addition to moving the patient frequently, see "Wounds."

Walk, walk, walk to prevent leg ulcers—and eat a diet high in vegetables and fruit. Forgo sweets altogether. If you have varicose veins, put up your feet when you sit. But walking is better than sitting.

Urinary Tract Infection (UTI)

Urinary tract infections occur mostly in women because of their shorter urethras. If a woman comes into my office and declares she has a UTI, she most likely is right. Sometimes other diseases can mimic a UTI—like vaginitis, interstitial cystitis, kidney problems, kidney and bladder stones, and food allergies—so it is a good idea to confer with your doctor.

Here's what you can do at home:

- Drink plenty of fluid. Cranberry juice diluted and unsweetened is best. (Avoid other juices altogether.)
- Don't hold your urine—follow the urge.
- Stop all sugar and white starches (they are feeding the bacteria), artificial sweeteners, dyes, alcohol and coffee.
- Avoid dairy.
- Blueberries are fighting infections with their blue color. Always have some frozen blueberries in your freezer. You can make a hot soup from frozen blueberries (see page 135).
- Stick to the healthful diet based on vegetables and fruit that I recommend (see chapter 8).
- Wash your private parts twice a day with water only.
- For personal hygiene, always wipe from the front to the back after a bowel movement (and teach this to little girls!).
- Wear underwear with a cotton crotch because modern fibers can lead to high humidity and warmth that further bacterial growth.
- Avoid personal douches; they might destroy your healthy vaginal flora and set you up for bad bacteria.
- Avoid diaphragms and spermicidals.

- Exercise. Walking and rowing, for instance, increase blood flow to the pelvic area, thus creating a healthier environment. (They also exercise your "sexual" muscles). All exercise will help you fight infections.
- Laugh. Laughing massages the belly, including your pelvic floor.

UTIs are more common in sexually active women. This is what you can do for prevention:

- Have sex only after you are nice and wet—or use a personal lubricant like K-Y Jelly.
- Menopausal women might also benefit from "female herbs"—see Hot Flashes and Other Menopausal Symptoms.
- Urinate before and right after sex to flush out bacteria.
- Ask your partner to be clean, especially behind his foreskin.
- Some women get UTIs from sitting in a bathtub. Switch to showers instead.

Have these herbs at hand and take them with the first signs of UTI:

- Echinacea
- Horsetail

- Usnea
- Uva ursi

Don't take them longer than a week before you see your doctor. If you experience fever or flank (the area of the back of your waist) pain, you need immediate attention from a physician.

Vaginal Dryness and Itching After Menopause

We now know that menopausal symptoms don't go away "all by themselves" as (male) doctors have assumed previously. So we have to cope. Here's what you can do:

- Apply vaginal jelly copiously.
- Take tinctures of black cohosh, red clover, wild yam and ginkgo, one dropper each in hot water every day, once or twice a day.
- Before taking artificial hormones, if you are having really bad symptoms, make yourself knowledgeable about natural (bioidentical) hormones—and insist that your doctor learn about them, too.

Varicose Veins

Varicose veins are widening vessels, usually in your legs. The big ones can look like twisted cords;

the tiny ones are also called spiderwebs. You can also get varicosities in other parts of your body. Hemorrhoids are varicose veins around and in your anus; men get varicoceles at the scrotum. There is probably a genetic base as to why the vessel walls give, but pregnancy, childbirth and long hours standing can worsen the condition. Most of the time it is only a cosmetic problem, but the large veins can erode and bleed, become infected and, worst of all, deep veins can clot, giving you a thrombosis that can be life-threatening. With any swelling and unexplained pains in your legs you should see a physician.

Do you want a surgical solution? I would not go under the knife for cosmetic reasons—only for medical ones. Try these things first:

- Walking pushes stagnant blood out of the vessels, so do not just stand around. If you have to stand, make tiny steps on the spot to activate the vein "pump" in your legs.
- Any exercise is beneficial for your veins, not only for activating the vein pump, but also by removing lysosomal enzymes that play a role in the development of the condition.
- Lose weight if you are too heavy. Fat in your abdominal area hinders the blood returning

from the legs to the heart by clamping off the vessels.

- A diet high in vegetables, fruit, berries and herbs will provide rutin and other flavonoids (a kind of antioxidant) that strengthen vessel walls.
- Bilberry extract, onions and garlic are top of the list for vein sufferers.
- Put up your legs when you sit.
- Don't cross your legs; that hinders blood flow.
- Wear support hose at all times. Preferably put them on in bed in the morning—not necessarily the medical kind, but some that keep the tissue together.
- Walk barefoot in cold water like in a creek or at the beach as often as you can.
- Avoid high heels.
- Take a cold shower after each warm one.
- Avoid hot or warm baths.
- Bromelain reduces the thick fibrin deposits around varicosities—at least in some people. Fresh pineapple is high in bromelain.
- Horse chestnut has a compound, aescin, that strengthens the vessel walls and makes them more elastic.
- Gotu kola reduces swelling by strengthening

the adhesive that holds the veins together.
- Take dried violet flowers as a tea—or their main compound, rutin, directly as a capsule. Buckwheat is another plant high in rutin that will strengthen your vessel walls.

After varicose vein surgery—called stripping— the surgeon will recommend you walk several miles per day to keep up the good result, so I would try to walk, walk, walk first—and postpone an invasive operation perhaps indefinitely.

Wrinkles
(See also Chapter 7, Look Good, Feel Good)

The skin mirrors what is going on inside your body—and it tells the story of your whole life. The happier you look, the less important a few crinkles will become. Smile at yourself in the mirror.

It never hurts to go on a cleansing regimen. Here are some cleansing herbs—take them daily for a month at a time as prescribed on the bottle:

- Dandelion
- Milk thistle
- Stinging nettle

I don't think that bowel cleansing programs are such a good idea—after all, what is *natural* about filling you up with a gallon of water from your rear end?

A good idea is a **fasting day** once a month. Try it over a weekend: Start with a light vegetarian dinner on Friday night. On Saturday have nothing but water and vegetable broth (throw into water as many vegetables and herbs you can put your hands on and boil for at least half an hour with a pinch of salt). Sip the *broth only* (no solids!) whenever you feel faint or hungry. Go for a walk at least once on that day. Light yoga is excellent, too. Next morning, start with a healthful breakfast (see chapter 8), and cook a soup or a stir-fry without meat or poultry. Pass the whole Sunday on a vegetarian fare.

Let the fasting be the beginning of a healthier lifestyle—not vegetarian, but definitely without dairy and with less meats and poultry.

Having said that the inside is more important in dealing with wrinkles, I admit that I use some cream on the outside anyway. Here is what works for me:

- **Pearlcream.** This is an affordable Chinese brand of cream; you get it in Chinese markets or pharmacies. I use Pearlcream around my eyes and on wrinkles in the face. (And, no, no one pays me to advertise their product. I have a deep respect for the thousands of years of wisdom in Traditional Chinese Medicine.)

- **Olive oil.** For the rest of my body, especially my neck, I use olive oil, sometimes with a few drops of essential oil (myrrh, oregano and thyme are my favorites) mixed in. Olive oil is wonderful against itching skin. Unlike petroleum-based lotions, it does not require more and more to work. And yes, I use the same olive oil I use in the kitchen.

Obviously, if you are displeased with your looks, the possibility of cosmetic surgery is always open to you—liposuction, botox injection and the like—but don't expect advice here from an integrative physician. During the years, I have seen some good results, but unfortunately I've seen my share of botched procedures, too. My philosophy is: Avoid unnecessary operations at all cost. Always get a second opinion. Try natural methods first.

RESOURCES

For more information about alternative/complementary practices, see Weisman, R. and Berman, B. *Own Your Health: Choosing the Best from Alternative & Conventional Medicine.* Deerfield Beach, Fla.: Health Communications, Inc., 2003.

Alexander Technique

Alexander Technique International
Web site: *www.ati-net.com*

Cancer

Memorial Sloan-Kettering Cancer Center
Web site: *www.mskcc.org/mskcc/html/11570.cfm*

National Cancer Institute
Web site: *www.cancer.gov*

Complementary and Alternative Medicine (CAM)

CAM on PubMed
Web site: *www.nlm.nih.gov/nccam/camonpubmed.html*

ClinicalTrials.Gov
Web site: *www.clinicaltrials.gov*

Combined Health Information Database (CHID)
Web site: *http://chid.nih.gov*

**The National Center for Complementary and
Alternative Medicine (NCCAM)**
Web site: *http://nccam.nih.gov*

**The National Center for Complementary and
Alternative Medicine (NCCAM) Public
Information Clearinghouse**
P.O. Box 7923
Gaithersburg, MD 20898
Phone: 1-888-644-6226; outside U.S.: (301) 519-3153
Fax: 1-866-464-3616 (Toll-Free)
TTY: 1-866-464-3615 (Toll-Free)
E-mail: *info@nccam.nih.gov*
Web site: *http://nccam.nih.gov/health/clearinghouse/index.htm*

Elder Abuse

The National Center on Elder Abuse
1201 15th Street, N.W., Suite 350
Washington, DC 20005
Phone: (202) 898-2586
Fax: (202) 898-2583
E-mail: *ncea@nsua.org*
Web site: *www.elderabusecenter.org/default.cfm*

Eye Health

National Eye Institute
Web site: *www.nei.nih.gov/news/pressreleases/032002.asp*

Herbs and Herbal Medicine

American Botanical Council
Web site: *www.herbalgram.org*

Berkeley Wellness Letter
Web site: *www.wellnessletter.com/html/ds/dsSupplements.php*

Columbia University
Web site: *www.rosenthal.hs.columbia.edu/Botanicals.html*

Council for Responsible Nutrition
Web site: *www.crnusa.org*

Herb Research Foundation
Web site: *www.herbs.org*

Herbal Materia Medica
Web site: *www.healthy.net/clinic/therapy/herbal/herbic/herbs*

McMaster University
Web site: *www-hsl.mcmaster.ca/tomflem/altmed.html*

National Center for Complementary and Alternative Medicine (Herbal Supplements)
Web site: *www.nccam.nih.gov/health/supplement-safety*

Natural Medicine Comprehensive Database (Subscription)
Web site: *www.naturaldatabase.com/(kwiy5045xskn3y45 dqcyq145)/home.aspx?li=0&st=0&cs=&s=ND*

Office of Dietary Supplements
Web site: *http://dietary-supplements.info.nih.gov/Health_ Information/IBIDS.aspx*

University of Pittsburgh
Web site: *www.pitt.edu/~cbw/database.html*

Publications

Duke, James A. *The Green Pharmacy*. Emmaus, PA: Rodale, 1997.

Garland, Sarah. *The Herb Garden*. New York: Penguin USA, 1996.

Levy, Juliette deBairacli. *Common Herbs for Natural Health*. Woodstock, NY: Ash Tree Publishing, 1997.

———. *Nature's Children*. New York: Warner Paperback Library, 1997.

McCaleb, Robert, Evelyn Leigh and Krista Morien. *The Encyclopedia of Popular Herbs*. Roseville, CA: Prima Health, 2000.

Murray, Michael T. *The Healing Power of Herbs: The Enlightened Person's Guide to the Wonders of Medicinal Plants*. Roseville, CA: Prima Publishing, 1995.

Robbers, James E., and Varro E. Tyler. *Herbs of Choice: The Therapeutic Use of Phytomedicinals*. Binghamton, NY: Haworth Press, 1996.

Twitchell, Paul. *Herbs: The Magic Healers: The Complete Guide to Physical and Spiritual Well-Being*. Eckankar Books.

Tyler, Varro E. *The Honest Herbal*. Binghamton, NY: Haworth Press, 1993.

Pain

American Chronic Pain Association
P.O. Box 850
Rocklin, CA 95677
E-mail: ACPA@pacbell.net
Web site: www.theacpa.org

American Pain Foundation
111 South Calvert Street, Suite 2700
Baltimore, MD 21202
Web site: www.painfoundation.org

Stress Management and Meditation

Publications

Bera, T., M. Gore and J. Oak. "Recovery from Stress in Two Different Postures and in Shavasana—A Yogic

Relaxation Posture." *Indian J Physiol Pharmacol* 42.4 (1998): 473–478.

Carrington, P. "The Physiology of Meditation." R. Woolfolk, eds. *Principles and Practice of Stress Management*. 2nd ed. New York: Guilford, 1993, 141.

Davidson, R. "Alterations in Brain and Immune Function Produced by Mindfulness Meditation." *Psychosom Med* 64.4 (2003): 564–570.

Jacobs, G. "The Physiology of Mind-Body Interactions: The Stress Response and the Relaxation Response. *J Altern Complement Med* 7(suppl. 1) (2001): S83–92.

Murugesan, R, N. Govindarajulu and T. Bera. "Effect of Selected Yogic Practices on the Management of Hypertension." *Indian J Physiol Pharmacol* 44.2 (2000): 207–210.

Raub, J. "Psychophysiologic Effects of Hatha Yoga on Musculoskeletal and Cardiopulmonary Function: A Literature Review." *J Alt Complementary Med* 8.6 (2002): 797–812.

Saraswati, S. S. *Yoga Nidra*, 6th ed. Bihar, India: Yoga Publications Trust, 1998.

Shannahoff-Khalsa, D. "An Introduction to Kundalini Yoga Meditation Techniques That Are Specific for the Treatment of Psychiatric Disorders." *J Altern Complement Med* 10.1 (2004): 91–101.

Yoga

The Yoga Site
Web site: *www.yogasite.com/articles.htm*
See article, "Why Do Yoga?" at
www.yogasite.com/why.htm.

YogaFinder (Finding a teacher)
Web site: *www.yogafinder.com*

Yoga Alliance
Web site: *www.yogaalliance.org/index.php*

Publications

Corliss, R. "The Power of Yoga." *Time* 157: 54–62.

Koertge, J., et al. "Improvement in Medical Risk Factors and Quality of Life in Women and Men with Coronary Artery Disease in the Multicenter Lifestyle Demonstration Project." *Am J Cardiol* 91.11 (2003): 1316–1322.

NOTES

1. Ester Shapiro, *Grief as a Family Process: A Cultural and Developmental Approach to Integrative Practice*, 2nd edition (New York: Guilford, in press).

2. Thomas T. Perls and Margery Hutter Silver, *Living to 100, Lessons in Living to Your Maximum Potential at Any Age* (New York: Basic Books, 1999).

3. Ibid., 63.

4. The hardiness research of Dr. Salvatore Maddi was described in the Samueli Institute Optimal Healing Environments initiative and research program in 2005. Referenced here with permission of Dr. Maddi and of the Samueli Institute.

5. Interviews with Salvatore R. Maddi, September 2005; S. R. Maddi, "Hardiness Training at Illinois Bell Telephone," in J. P. Opatz, ed., *Health Promotion Evaluation* (Stevens Point, WI: National Wellness Institute, 1987), 101–115; and S. R. Maddi, "The Story of Hardiness: Twenty Years of Theorizing, Research and Practice," *Consulting Psychology Journal: Practice and Research* 54 (2002): 173–185.

6. S. C. Kobasa, S. R. Maddi and S. Kahn, "Hardiness and Health: A Prospective Study," *Journal of Personality and Social Psychology* 42 (1982): 884–890.

7. S. C. Kobasa et al., "Relative Effects of Hardiness, Exercise and Social Support as Resources Against Illness," *Journal of Psychosomatic Research* 29 (1986): 525–533.

8. For more information about hardiness training programs: Hardiness Institute, 4199 Campus Drive, Suite 550, Irvine, CA 92612; phone: (949) 252-0580; fax: (949) 252-8087; e-mail: *hardiness1@aol.com*; Web site: *www.hardinessinstitute.com*.

9. D. M. Khoshaba and S. R. Maddi, *HardiTraining* (Newport Beach, CA: Hardiness Institute, 2001).

10. Dr. Pennebaker's research was described in the Samueli Institute Optimal Healing Environments initiative and research program in

2005. Referenced here with permission of the Samueli Institute. For more information, see J. Pennebaker, *Writing to Heal: A Guided Journal for Recovering from Trauma and Emotional Upheaval* (Oakland, CA: New Harbinger Press, 2004).

11. J. Pennebaker, *Writing to Heal: A Guided Journal for Recovering from Trauma and Emotional Upheaval* (Oakland, CA: New Harbinger Press, 2004); and J. Pennebaker, *Opening Up: The Healing Power of Expressing Emotions*, revised edition (New York: Guilford Press, 1997).

12. M. Van Willigen, "Differential Benefits of Volunteering Across the Life Course," *Journals of Gerontology: Series B: Psychological Sciences & Social Sciences* 55B (2000): S308–S318.

13. T. Field, "Elder Retired Volunteers Benefit from Giving Massage Therapy to Infants," *J Appl Gerontol* 17 (1998): 229–239.

14. S. O'Laoire, "An Experimental Study of the Effects of Distant, Intercessory Prayer on Self-Esteem, Anxiety, and Depression," *Altern Ther Health Med* 3.6 (November 1997): 38–53; and J. A. Dusek et al., "Healing Prayer Outcomes Studies: Consensus Recommendations," *Altern Ther Health Med* 9.3 (suppl.) (May–Jun 2003): A44–53.

15. Deepak Chopra, *Ageless Body, Timeless Mind: The Quantum Alternative to Growing Old* (New York: Harmony, 1994).

16. J. T. Cacioppo and L. C. Hawkley, "Social Isolation and Health, with an Emphasis on Underlying Mechanisms," *Perspect Biol Med* 46.3 (suppl.) (2003): S39–52; and B. Justice, *Who Gets Sick: How Beliefs, Moods and Thoughts Affect Health* (Houston, TX: Peak Press, 2000).

17. I. S. Wittstein et al., "Neurohumoral Features of Myocardial Stunning Due to Sudden Emotional Stress," *N Engl J Med* 352.6 (2005): 539–548.

18. Lynda W. Freeman, *Best Practices in Complementary and Alternative Medicine: An Evidence-Based Approach with Nursing CE/CME* (Gaithersburg, MD: Aspen Publishers, 2001), 8-1:1.

19. Fred Luskin, *Forgive for Good* (New York: HarperCollins, 2002), xv.

20. Ibid.

21. Ibid., 68.

22. Telephone interview with Dr. Fred Luskin by Roanne Weisman, April 23, 2002.

23. Luskin, op. cit. 211.

24. Telephone interview with Dr. Fred Luskin by Roanne Weisman, April 23, 2002.

25. Telephone interview with Dr. Fred Luskin by Roanne Weisman, April 23, 2002.

26. Helen Nearing, *Loving and Leaving the Good Life* (New York: Chelsea Green Publishing Company, 1993).

27. Sogyal Rinpoche, *The Tibetan Book of Living and Dying* (San Francisco: HarperSanFrancisco, 1994).

28. Duke Center for Integrative Medicine SEARCH Study: "Support, Education and Research in Chronic Heart Failure," *www. dukemagazine.duke.edu/dukemag/issues/091002/health-heart.html*.

29. Norman Cousins, *Anatomy of an Illness* (New York: Bantam, 1981), 39.

30. Ibid., 86.

31. Patient interview by Roanne Weisman, Spring 1999.

32. S. Wolf et. al., "Reducing Frailty and Falls in Older Persons: An Investigation of Tai Chi and Computerized Balance Training," *Journal of American Geriatric Society* 44 (1996): 489–497.

33. L. Wolfson et. al., "Balance and Strength Training in Older Adults: Intervention Gains and Tai Chi Maintenance," *Journal of American Geriatric Society* 44 (May 1996): 498–506.

34. S. S. Haas, "Hydrotherapy and More: Adapting Kneipp's Natural Medicine to the U.S.," *Complementary Medicine for the Physician* 5.8 (2000): 57, 61–64.

35. Reprinted with permission from James A. Duke, from the Website: *http://wavefunctioncollapse.blogspot.com/2005/08/dukes-geriatric-dozen.html*; originally appeared in *Dr. Duke's Essential Herbs* (Emmaus, PA: Rodale, 1999).

36. B. Berman et al., "Effectiveness of Acupuncture as Adjunctive Therapy in Osteoarthritis of the Knee: A Randomized Controlled Trial," *Ann Intern Med* 141 (2004): 901–910.

37. Kenneth Pelletier, *The Best Alternative Medicine: What Works? What Does Not?* (New York: Simon & Shuster, 2000), 324–326.

38. James A. Duke, *The Green Pharmacy* (Emmaus, PA: Rodale, 1997), 55.

39. Ibid.

40. S. Wolf et al., "Reducing Frailty and Falls in Older Persons: An Investigation of Tai Chi and Computerized Balance Training," *Journal of American Geriatric Society* 44 (1996): 489–497.

41. L. Wolfson et.al., "Balance and Strength Training in Older Adults: Intervention Gains and Tai Chi Maintenance," *Journal of American Geriatric Society* 44 (May 1996): 498–506.

42. Laura Lewis, *52 Ways to Live a Long and Healthy Life* (New York: MJF Books, 1993).

43. Fuzhong Li et al., "Improving Physical Function and Blood Pressure in Older Adults Through Cobblestone Mat Walking: A Randomized Trial," *Journal of the American Geriatrics Society* 53.8 (2005): 1305–1312.

ABOUT THE AUTHORS

Alexa Fleckenstein, M.D., of Whole Health New England, is a physician, teacher, writer, inspirational speaker, gardener and mother. She is board-certified in Internal Medicine, with training in Germany and the United States. She also holds a subspecialty degree in Natural Medicine from Germany. She has a special interest in wellness and rejuvenation, particularly the healing effects of water. As an integrative physician in the Boston area, she has taken care of patients in clinics and hospitals for more than twenty years and gives frequent workshops in integrative medicine for community health organizations and in corporate settings.

Roanne Weisman writes in the areas of science, medicine and health care. She is the principal author of the award-winning book, *Own Your Health: Choosing the Best from Alternative & Conventional Medicine* (HCI Books 2003). Her articles and feature stories have appeared in newspapers as well as in *Alternative Medicine Magazine*, *Body & Soul Magazine* and *Country Living Magazine*. She also writes extensively for the publications of most of the teaching hospitals of the Harvard Medical School. She has spoken and conducted workshops around the U.S. and in Canada on integrative medicine, which include her personal story of how "owning" her health helped her recover from a paralyzing stroke.